THE
WAY
SHE
WEARS
IT

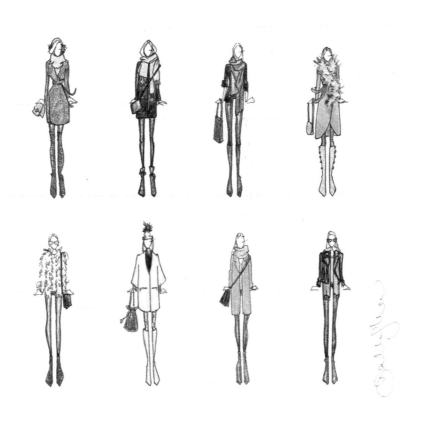

WILLIAM MORROW

An Imprint of HarperCollins*Publishers*

THE WAY SHE WEARS IT

the ultimate insider's guide to revealing your personal style

DALLAS SHAW

HarperCollins books may be purchased for educational, business, or sales promotional use. For information please e-mail the Special Markets Department at SPsales@harpercollins.com.

FIRST EDITION

Designed by Suet Yee Chong
Photography by Alison Conklin
Illustrations by Dallas Shaw
Styled by Beka Rendell

Library of Congress Cataloging-in-Publication Data
has been applied for.

ISBN 978-0-06-245546-8

17 18 19 20 21 LSCC 10 9 8 7 6 5 4 3 2 1

This book is dedicated to
the entire staff at
LaSalle the Image Makers.

love you.
mean it.

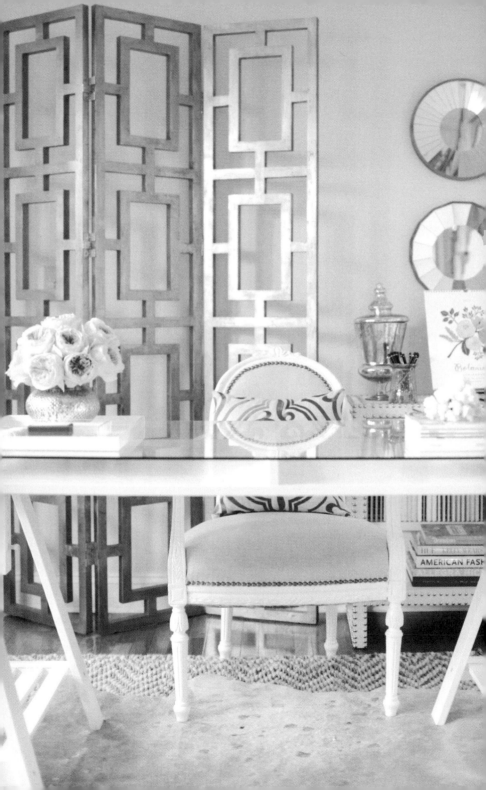

CONTENTS

<u>ch.</u> 04 SUMMER 89

<u>ch.</u> 05 FALL 137

ᶜʰ· 06 WINTER 193

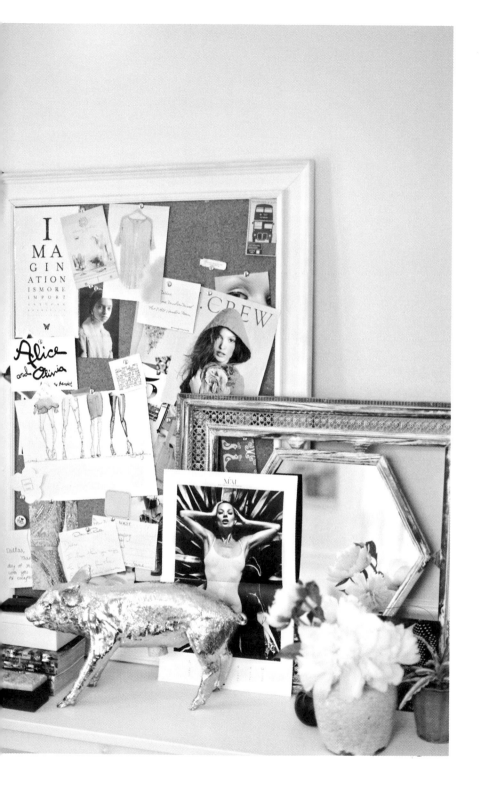

you

know

who

she is

She walks into a room and everyone notices. People wonder—
and some even ask—"Who is that girl?" She exudes confidence in her
subtle movements, her red lip, and the sparkle in her eye. She smiles
and immediately has all eyes on her. She's not just well dressed;
she's magnetic.

She makes you rethink your own fashion rules and she makes you
want to break them. She has just the right watch for the
silk shirt, just the right mules for her perfectly tailored jeans that
show just the right amount of ankle. She intrigues you, and everyone
else around you, with the way her dress delicately kisses the floor as
she sweeps across the room.

Her clothing palette is a mix of unexpected color and
looks effortless. Rhinestones with plaid, lace with leather,
neon with pastels. It's not the jacket she's wearing;
it's the way she wears it.

And when she leaves the room, she's still on everyone's
mind because the scent of her signature perfume lingers
in the air.

SHE IS YOU.

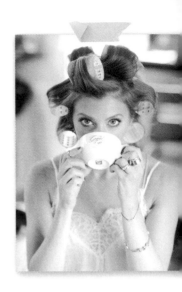

INTRODUCTION

We have all seen the woman from the previous page, and we all long to be her. And I'm here to show you how.

I have spent the last decade making a name for myself as an illustrator and project designer in the fashion industry.

I wake up at five thirty A.M. and run around in heels until eleven thirty P.M. or until my eyelids simply can't stay open to look at visual concepts a single second longer. After I draw with designers, I hang out a bit to weigh in on shoes and accessories. Then I talk hemlines and color. Last week I actually had an hour-and-a-half-long meeting to discuss a bike basket. True story. I spend my hours sketching, painting, designing, (coffee here) pulling palettes, searching beautiful imagery, scribbling on mood boards with giant "X's" and equally giant "YES!!'s" (more coffee here). I'm often running from show to show, working on design collaborations, drawing collections, sitting in on top-secret board meetings, sharing my personal style tips with powerhouse brands, previewing collections in designer showrooms, explaining how color matching works and why I am responding to visuals.

To sum it up, I spend every waking hour of my career surrounded by beautiful things and creative geniuses—and I've been taking serious notes. In between the double cheek kisses and coffee runs, I've learned a thing or two about personal style. Designers have liked my artwork, but they always want something more: to know about my personal taste. Designers don't only hire me for my creativity—they hire me because I *am* their target market, and I know exactly what I like and why I like it. I can attend nearly any event feeling comfortable and confident in my style.

But it took me a while to reach that point. The key was challenging myself to stop dressing for others and begin dressing for myself. I learned what I liked, why I liked it, and, most important, what made me feel comfortable and confident. I learned that not all trends suit my style, and that some unexpected trends became all-time favorites. And now I have taken everything I learned along the way and created this personal fashion journey. It's a lookbook-meets-workbook organized into challenges I created just for you.

Whether you're a self-proclaimed fashion novice who's easing in, a fashionista who wants to step up her game, or the most stylish one in the room already (which you stay on top of by keeping up with

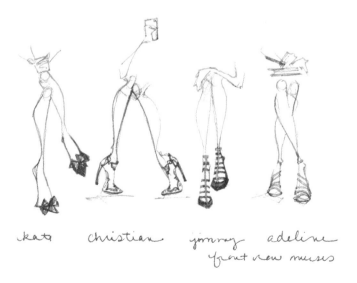

kate   christian   jimmy   adeline
your new muses

expert picks like the ones in this book), I wrote this book for you. Along with the challenges, I'll bust fashion myths, share insider industry tricks, but above all else, I hope I'll inspire you to live beautifully. After completing the style challenges in this book, you, the reader, will have rebranded yourself.

We'll work together to mix up the pieces you already own, figure out how to let your personality shine with color pairings, and even cover how to pull off the "unexpected" in your daily life (without looking like a circus act). I've brought notes, photos, and inspiration. I've sharpened my pencils, broken out my art supplies, and cleared my schedule for a bit. I'll meet you in the closet.

x/

Dallas Shaw

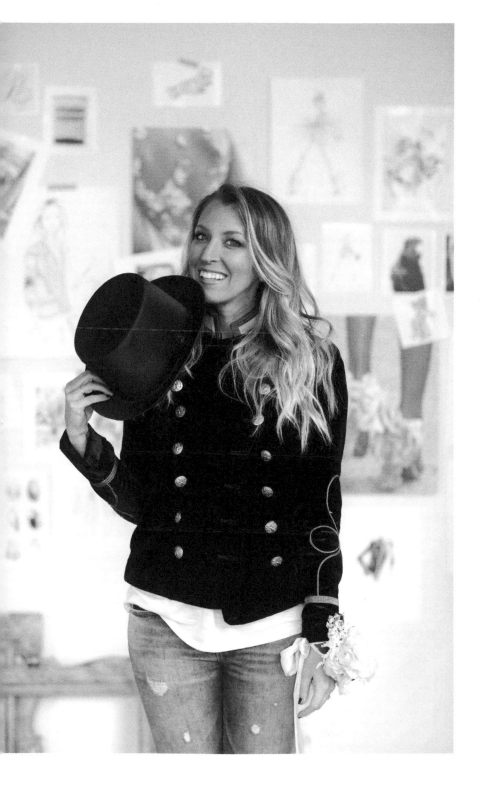

How to Use This Book

Remember when personal style seemed so much easier? Didn't things seem more simplified when people could just match their clothes and fit into a specific fashion category like "classic" or "minimalist"? Why did everyone have to start mixing things up and looking so good?

Street-style photographs and bloggers emerged everywhere, and whether you loved it or hated it, along with them came a raised awareness that fashion was—yet again—about to mix things up. The way that real girls, not celebrities with stylists, were piecing high-end and low-end items together was refreshing. Women suddenly wanted to match less and complement more, which in turn complicated things for shoppers everywhere. Even fashion pros started becoming more thoughtful about print pairings and accessory placement, making it nearly impossible to keep up with the flood of inspirational style imagery surrounding us.

In the past, personal style was easier to choose than to understand. It's no longer about checking a classic/bohemian/casual/trendy box and choosing items only from that box for the rest of your life. No more living in fashion boxes! This book will break the rules of style categories and help you understand what you feel best in. This is a visual guide to finding your own personal style through a set of beautiful prompts. By the end of this book you'll be confident in your own stylish skin and you'll feel comfortable dressing for everything from the office to the front row of fashion shows.

If you take some time to truly understand your personal style, you can clear up a lot of space in your closet and—bonus—clear out a lot of chaos in your life. You'll have a better understanding of who you are. You'll own less "stuff" and more treasures. You'll save money by purchasing only the items you know you'll wear. Don't panic: You won't have to stop shopping—you'll just shop smarter. Most important, you'll be happy because you'll genuinely live in your unique personal style.

By purchasing this book, you're making a pact to do two things, with me as your guide:

1. Try new things.
2. Try new things on.

You will be trying new techniques before you know it, and with each new style challenge, I'd like you to reflect on how you felt about it to find out why you do and don't like certain styles. Ask yourself "why" often. Understanding *why* things make you feel good is the key to progressing in this journey. This is a style self-awareness book. Uncovering and investigating your likes and dislikes will help to bring out your improved self.

warning: you will be challenged.

It's not easy to determine your own style. How many times have you felt confident that you have finally found your authentic look only to stare blankly at your closet one week later? (Hi. Me, biweekly.) If you use this book as intended, I promise you you'll finally figure it out so you can begin to feel great and look your very best every day.

By purchasing this book, you are about to embark on a style journey, and somewhere along the way you will come out with a clear understanding of your own personal style and a more confident version of yourself.

why you need this book

Your style is important. A first impression is made within the first seven seconds of meeting someone. SEVEN seconds. Which means by the time you finish reading this sentence, I've already decided whether I can trust you based on your appearance right now. Scary.

This is exactly why your style should reflect your personality. It's an extension of your own personal brand and deserves some attention and care. We're going to get you to the point where your style is so spot-on that they only need three of those seven seconds to know exactly who you are.

What image are you projecting at this very moment? Are you confident, or could you use a bit of self-reinvention?

Post: This book isn't really about how good you'll look; it's about how good you'll feel.

Not to worry—you can begin at any moment, so why not right now? Make the decision to give the challenges in this book a shot as a form of self-care. It's simple. Once you make the decision and the commitment to embrace a new more stylish life, you can start living that life immediately.

Q: *What if you already know your own style and just need some new inspiration?*
A: *Good news: You can use this book for general clothing ruts, too.*

This book is for the shoe shoppers. The fashion lovers. Those of us whose closets could use a bit of breathing room. Use this book if you are looking to become more adventurous in your personal style, or if you're a fashionista who needs a refresh—not necessarily of your wardrobe but of your interest in your current wardrobe. The outcome for both is to embrace your clothes and stop spending money on things you wear only once. Or nonce.

Following a set of rules when it comes to clothing, copying off of celebs or store mannequins will get you dressed but won't bring you joy. Let's have some fun with this!

all that, and . . .

{ what else will this book do? }

CHANGE THE WAY YOU SHOP

Retail therapy exists but doesn't produce long-term results unless you understand what you are shopping for and why you're shopping. I shop often. I do it for the thrill of the hunt. The entire process is relaxing for me. When you know your style, you begin to understand what you wear most and why, and in turn you will "want" less. The desire to spend aimlessly fades away and you naturally begin to shop smarter. I'm all for spending more on the things you truly love and will live in. By learning about your personal style you will invest more in those "forever pieces."

TEACH YOU TO TRUST YOUR TASTE

In the past you may have gone into a store and trusted an employee to tell you what to wear and buy, and in doing so, have taken on their personal style instead of yours. You've also probably let friends talk you in or out of items. From now on, you have to believe that you can figure it out for yourself. This book is about finding your own personal style, designing a new and improved lifestyle, and viewing your clothing as a reflection of yourself—don't start by wearing another person's style.

GIVE YOU THE TOOLS TO SHOP SMARTER

Everyone has a "thing," and mine is clothes. It didn't hit me that I was buying the same items over and over again until a few years ago. I was working in fashion, so I was surrounded by clothes all the time and shopping a lot. Working through these challenges on my own, and learning to stop and ask "Why do I like this?" has changed my life and my bank account. Knowing the "why" helped me understand my spending on a deeper level. I now know my style well enough to know that I'll buy anything with birds on it. I swipe my card at any combination of pink and red. Gold sequins are my weakness. By the end of

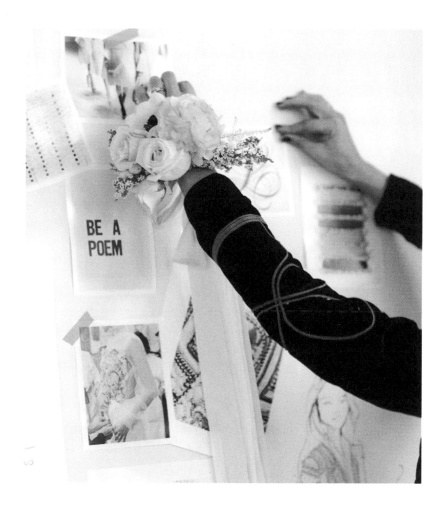

this book you'll be asking yourself the question "What do I like about this?" regularly, and it will empower you to make more strategic purchases.

One of the best things that comes with knowing your style? It doesn't take nearly as long to get ready in the morning, and you will once and for all cut out the inevitable closet-full-of-nothing-to-wear dance.

{ what you'll see as you go }

REFLECTION PROMPTS

I'd like you to learn what you like and why you like it. These prompts will ask you to reflect on what you like about the challenge. How did it make you feel and why? What would you change about the look next time to feel even better in it or to make it more your own?

MINI CHALLENGES

Throughout the book you'll find a series of mini challenges for the over-achievers. These will push you even further by keeping you extra style-savvy and organized.

DS FAVES

I keep a long mental list of favorites at every lifestyle brand and can rattle them off like Rain Man, so if you can keep up with me, you'll find some under DS faves throughout the book and a longer list at the back of the book.

TIPS ✕

Top-secret tips and tricks of the trade I've learned from spending years with the best in the business.

#THINGSWENEED

This one is self-explanatory.

THERAPY CHECK-INS

Every so often in this book you will come across a pink page that will prompt you to think about how you are doing. Be honest with yourself and your answers here. If you aren't feeling a challenge, think about why and try it differently in a more authentic way until you feel good about yourself. The goal is to get you to a place where you can answer positively about your fashion and beauty adventures. It's not just about the clothes—it's about your whole look and how it makes you feel.

Therapy Sesh

Before we get to the challenges, I'd like to ask you to do some careful consideration of your image. While you might want to skip right to the closet, order is important in your new life (which starts right now), so we'll need to start at the beginning for all this to work. Welcome to your much-needed therapy session. Here we go.

Imagine your most stylish you. The style-icon you. You, on your most confident and put-together day. Close your eyes, take a bath, deep breathing, whatever you need to do to relax, and think about this. Really try to envision that stylish you as someone else notices you from across the room. You're smiling and happy and others come up to you mid—champagne sip and say, "I'm so sorry to interrupt but I have to know where you got that clutch." Valentino—but back to the dream: I'm going to need you to do whatever is needed to channel that version of yourself. Take time with this vision and get in touch with that girl.

When you are ready, answer the questions below:

1. DESCRIBE YOUR PERSONALITY IN FIVE WORDS.

   [1.] .... [4.] ....

   [2.] .... [5.] ....

   [3.] ....

2. DESCRIBE YOUR STYLE IN FIVE WORDS.

   [1.] .... [4.] ....

   [2.] .... [5.] ....

   [3.] ....

3. WHAT COLOR FEELS MOST TRUE TO YOUR PERSONAL STYLE?

   ....

   ....

4. WHAT IS YOUR HAIR COLOR AND STYLE, AND WHO/WHAT ORIGINALLY INSPIRED YOU TO GET THAT CUT?

5. WHAT COLOR LIP DO YOU WEAR ON A SPECIAL NIGHT OUT?

6. DESCRIBE YOUR FAVORITE ITEM IN YOUR CLOSET.

7. WHAT WAS THE VERY LAST ITEM YOU PURCHASED? WHEN YOU BOUGHT IT, WHAT OUTFIT WERE YOU ENVISIONING IT WOULD BE PERFECT WITH?

8. WHAT'S YOUR SIGNATURE PERFUME?

That felt good, right? Now comes the second part to this reflection. You may find this a bit challenging, but answer honestly. It's the only way to make progress.

1. LIST THE LAST THREE OUTFITS YOU WORE. TODAY, YESTERDAY, AND THE DAY BEFORE. NO NEED TO INCLUDE EXCUSES FOR WHAT YOU WORE "I WAS ONLY RUNNING ERRANDS SO—" STOP. JUST LIST. 1, 2, 3.

[1.]

[2.]

[3.]

2. LOOK AT THOSE THREE OUTFITS YOU LISTED. IF SOMEONE MET YOU FOR THE FIRST TIME IN THE PAST THREE DAYS, DO YOUR LOOKS REFLECT YOUR ANSWERS TO QUESTION 1 ON PAGE 15?

3. DO THOSE THREE LOOKS REFLECT YOUR ANSWERS TO QUESTION 2 ON PAGE 15?

4. DID YOU WEAR LIPSTICK THIS WEEK? .... TODAY? .... IF YOU DID, WAS IT THE SAME SHADE AS THE SHADE YOU SAID YOU'D WEAR ON A NIGHT OUT? ....

5. DID YOU STYLE YOUR HAIR TODAY? .... YESTERDAY? DID IT LOOK SIMILAR TO WHEN YOU LEFT THE SALON?

6. LET'S GO BACK TO YOUR FAVORITE ITEM IN YOUR CLOSET. HOW OFTEN DO YOU REALLY WEAR IT? DAILY? .... WEEKLY? .... DO YOU SAVE IT FOR SPECIAL OCCASIONS?

7. NOW LET'S GO BACK TO THE LAST ITEM YOU BOUGHT. HAVE YOU WORN IT YET? .... DID YOU WEAR IT WITH THE FULL INTENDED LOOK THAT YOU DREAMED UP IN YOUR MIND WHEN YOU PURCHASED IT? ....

8. DO YOU SPRAY YOUR SIGNATURE PERFUME AS PART OF YOUR MORNING ROUTINE? .... ARE YOU WEARING IT RIGHT NOW? ....

This concludes a little game I like to call "but, do you actually?" You get the point. The majority of us have a really beautiful vision of our personal style that lives in our minds but likely isn't actually being reflected in what we wear. And it doesn't make sense, because our closets are filled with things we *haaad to have*. We know what we like, we buy what we like, but most of us are not actually living our personal brand on a daily basis. Why the disconnect? What is stopping us from living that stylish story in our minds? It's not like we don't have the shoes to make it happen.

Here's the thing: it's normal. The second part of the reflection is a bit of a setback for 99 percent of us. (And that 1 percent of you . . . well, maybe you should write a book.) Don't feel bad about yourself. You're not an imposter. We are busy, really busy, and we don't have the time it takes to think about putting together the perfect look, so often when getting ready we opt to go the easy route. The problem is, the easy route isn't likely to project the best version of ourselves. And that is the very thing we are going to change in the following pages. By the end of this book, we'll get you to a place where all your clothing reflects your true style. And here's the best part—you'll figure it out all by yourself.

repeat after me:
"i'm going to begin living
in my personal style.
                    every. single. day."

{ what to know about the challenges }

Each challenge will prompt you to try something new, or to find renewed interest in overlooked pieces in your closet. Start your journey with the Prep (page 26), then go directly to the beginning of the season you are currently in. Your transformation will likely take a full year. If you are a beginner, you can use the book over and over again until you feel more adventurous. If you are already an expert, you can look to the book for new inspiration.

I can promise you this works. I was working in the lifestyle industry for six years when I felt like I'd had it up to here with people telling me all the things I "had" to do. How I should look to fit in with a company's style, how I should dress for social media posts, how I haaaad to stop smiling in photos (seriously?). The last straw was when a stylist told me I needed to wear all black to a meeting or I wouldn't get hired.

At that very moment, I decided to stop listening to everyone's advice and begin dressing exactly like I wanted to. Starting with that meeting. I wore a few colors and still got the gig. From that point on, I wore what made me feel best, and I took pride in getting dressed. I had a little fun with it and I even disobeyed the "rules" once in a while. That's when my career changed forever. Turns out, when I was dressed like me, I *felt* like my best me. My newfound confidence was evident. I was signing with larger companies; my rates tripled. I'm not sure what it is you are hoping for next in life, but if you figure out how to own your personal style, you might get a whole lot closer to those goals. In the end, it has nothing and everything to do with your clothes. Your spirit knows when you feel good.

things to remember as we get started

SECOND TIME'S A CHARM

Ever notice that the second time you wear a piece of clothing, it tends to look better than it did on the first wear? When you quickly throw an item on that second time, you aren't overthinking what to pair it with. Give each challenge a few tries and every item a few wears with different pairings before deciding on the combination that feels most "you."

GOOD DESIGN IS MEANT TO BE ENJOYED

Don't stow away your designer duds. Wear those things and wear them out. Mix those high-end pieces with low-end pieces and make them your own.

CREATE RENEWED INTEREST IN YOUR CLOSET

During each challenge, take a moment with each item of clothing and recall the newness and excitement you felt when you first made the purchase. Repurposing the clothes you already own will help you to appreciate them even more; plus, you'll spend less on new ones.

EACH CHALLENGE IS MEANT TO INSPIRE, NOT REQUIRE

Some of the items in this book cost thousands of dollars and other cost tens of dollars, and you won't know which because good design is good design no matter what the price tag. When I say diamonds, you can try cubic zirconia or even rhinestones. If I challenge you to wear pink and you don't own any pink, choose a different color you rarely wear, like yellow or emerald, instead. Gold can mean gold-plated and that is A-OK.

This book will bring out your best you. Are you ready to take the challenge? Let's get started!

{ confidence 101 }

LESSON 1: SMILE

The easiest way to convey confidence and a positive attitude, which will come in handy when trying new things.

LESSON 2: KNOW YOUR BODY

We are all made differently, and if a challenge suggests something that doesn't work for you, know that. Try it in your own way that flatters you and makes you feel unstoppable.

I very quickly want to address something important. This book is meant to be a visual inspiration. My fashion illustrations are stylized. They are long, leggy drawings, and they do not and in no way are supposed to reflect a natural body type. Drawings are not real. You are. This book exists for you to take this inspiration and create a masterpiece of your own.

LESSON 3: BREAK THE RULES

This is not a book of fashion rules—however, I do have one rule that you already agreed to in the pact we made on page 10: Try things on. There are certain cuts that complement certain body types and heights. A slight flare on a boot cut will flatter a tall figure. High-waisted denim looks amazing on somebody very petite. Does that mean somebody tall shouldn't wear high-waisted jeans? Not necessarily. Try it on to see how it looks on you.

{ style studies }

shopping lists

outfit notes

Let's begin our journey!
A few suggestions as we get
started:

TAKE NOTES

I suggest tracking your prog-
ress for yourself. Your call whether it's
notes in the margins of this book, a separate note-

reflections

book, or a brand-new planner. For me, being handed a new notebook
or planner is like being handed a new life. The fresh pages inspire a
new beginning, and I buy the most beautiful one each year so I can
start over with aspiration and organization. You plan all other important things in life, so take your new style seriously.

DO YOUR FASHION HOMEWORK

Find an hour of time tonight. Pour a glass of tea or wine, light a candle,
grab a laptop, put on some music, and log in to Pinterest. Create a secret pin board, begin scrolling through fashion images, and pin or save
the looks you love. Do this without overthinking. Do you love it? Save
it. At the end of the hour scroll through the images you saved. Here is
the starting point for your new look.

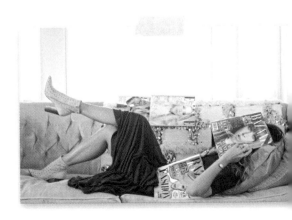

STUDY THOSE PUBLICATIONS

While there are countless forms of inspiration online, there is nothing like turning the pages of a beautiful publication like *Vogue* or *Harper's Bazaar*. Turning to trusted publications can help you figure out what you like if you don't have a clear vision yet. Fashion magazine research is my personal prep step. As you flip through the editorials, notice where your eye is stopping; is it a certain color combo that sparked your interest? That's called inspiration. Save that page.

L'OFFICIEL   N° 947 | AOÛT 2010

DECEMBER 2011   VOGUE

HARPER'S BAZAAR   OC

HARPER'S BAZAAR   FEBRUA

HARPER'S BAZAAR   JUN

HARPER'S BAZAAR FEBRUARY 2014

HARPER'S BAZAAR   JUN

SEPTEMBER 2013   VOGUE

VOGUE   N° 933   DÉCEMBRE 2012-JANVIER 2013

Meet Me in the Closet

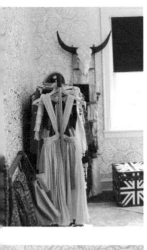
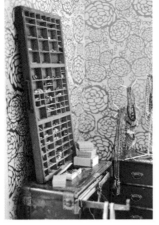
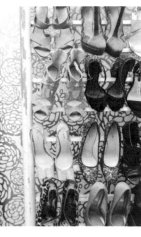
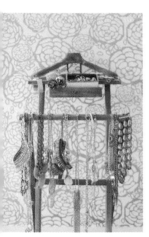
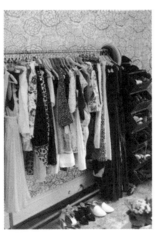
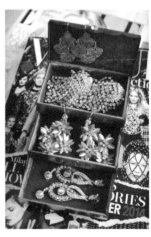
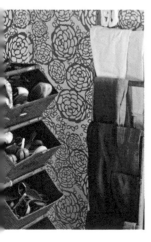
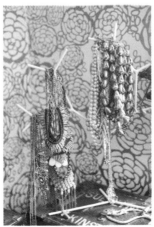
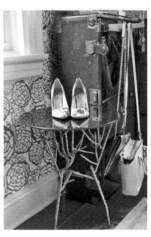

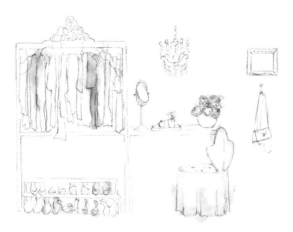

Now that you are feeling ready and excited, it's time for some quick closet prep. You'll be taking your clothing more seriously, so the place you store your clothes should be kept neat and organized as well.

#THINGSWENEED

A lint brush   A rolling rack
A sweater shaver   Wooden hangers
Scented drawer liners   Wrinkle release spray

 Wooden hangers are a wise investment. Take
care of those clothes.

The first commitment you'll be making is to take special care of your clothing, both on your body and on the hanger. Make sure to hang up each garment at the end of every night. I have a quiet Sunday night ritual where I neaten, steam, and brush the lint off everything. It helps me to appreciate every piece when they are hanging neatly in order.

✳ Be extra gentle when taking items on and off so as not to stretch, pull, or get makeup on them.

I have a thing for mohair, but I have to make sure that I remove any jewelry I'm wearing when taking mohair items off or putting them on.

As you are straightening up your closet, now is the time to get rid of any items you no longer need. #ThingsWeDon'tNeed: Anything that is ripped or stained, that no longer fits you in size, or that no longer fits your taste. Make a trip to Goodwill and make room in your closet only for what makes you feel great. Take the time to take care of this special space as you curate it over the next year.

✳ Keep a list of items that need replacing, or note this in your planner. It will help you stay focused during your next shopping trip.

While organizing today, think of unique ways to display your items. My denim hangs from an iron ladder, and an old piece of the window is my storage solution for shoes.

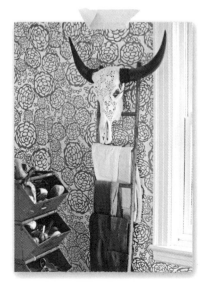

Back to BASICS

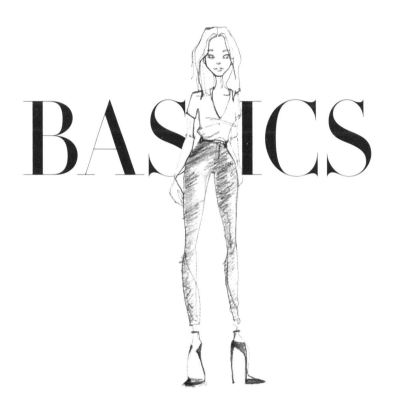

Basics are the foundation of a wardrobe and yet they tend to be the things we take for granted. Starting with T-shirts, they're what we buy most often and wear most often, but we often forget what an essential part of our wardrobe and life these tees are. Before we get started with the challenges, let's turn your focus to rebuilding your basics.

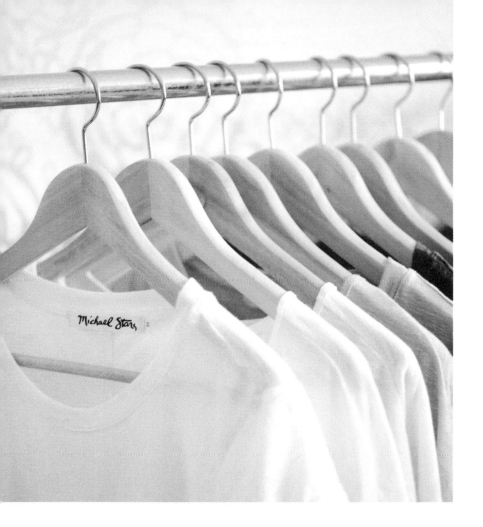

get started:

1. You don't need twenty mediocre white tees with different necklines; you only need one with an amazing fit.
2. Find your favorite style (it's actually fun to go out and only try on T-shirts) and invest in four or five different colors of the same shirt. I own the Michael Stars short-sleeved V-neck pocket tee in white, light gray, navy, dark gray, and cream and they hang in my closet in that order. These go-to essentials are my uniform, and I wear them with

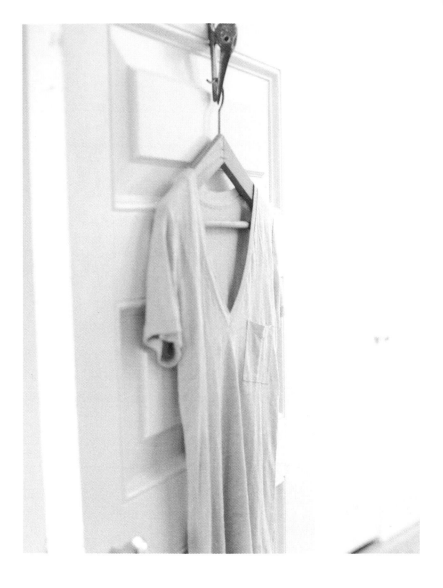

everything: jeans, pencil skirts, for Sunday lounging. With each wear—and that's a lotta wear—they look and feel that much cooler.

3. Ensure the correct fit. These tops should look easy and effortless. No one reading this book is allowed to wear baby tees, hear me? I often go one full size up on T-shirts. If they are too tight, they just look uncomfortable.

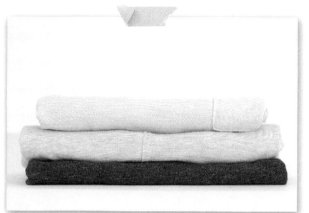

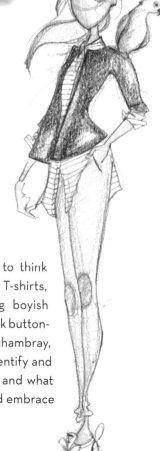

Once you've tackled your tees, it's time to think about your other basics. I personally love linen T-shirts, long-sleeved gray henleys (there's something boyish about them that I can't find in any other basic), silk button-downs, long-sleeved cashmere turtlenecks, chambray, and stripes. Lots of stripes. Take a minute to identify and go through your basics, deciding what to keep and what to replace. Steam them, hang them in order, and embrace them before moving forward.

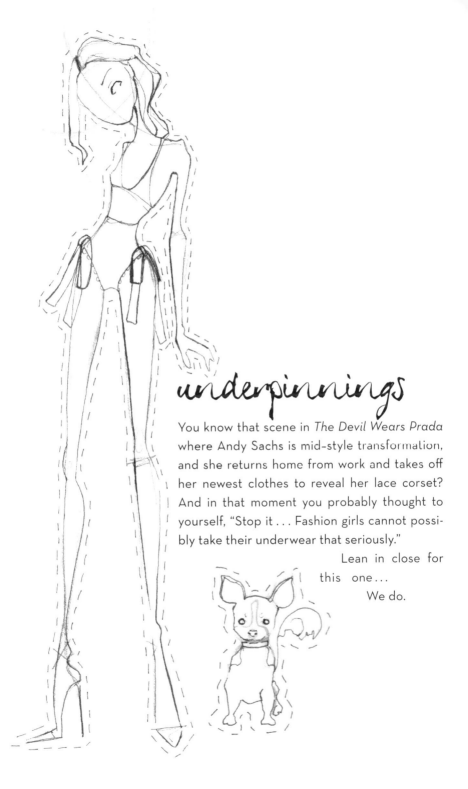

underpinnings

You know that scene in *The Devil Wears Prada* where Andy Sachs is mid-style transformation, and she returns home from work and takes off her newest clothes to reveal her lace corset? And in that moment you probably thought to yourself, "Stop it . . . Fashion girls cannot possibly take their underwear that seriously."

Lean in close for this one . . .

We do.

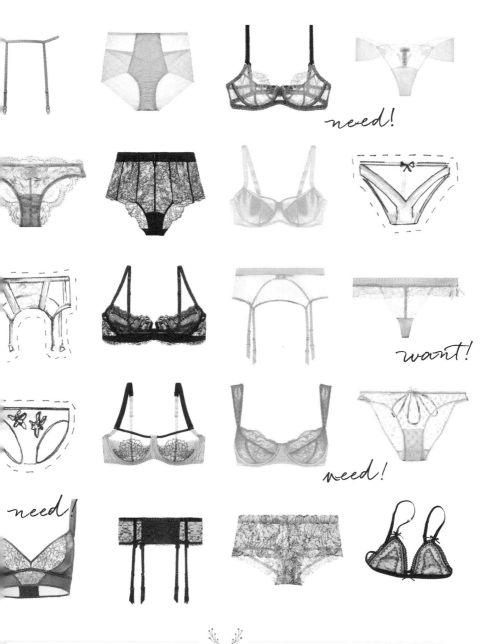

need!

want!

need!

need!

#THINGSWENEED

A lacy nude set for spring (not white—nude; you can see white through a white T-shirt, but you can't see nude) and an equally lacy black set for fall. Lace, ladies, you deserve that luxury. You can mix your other colors with these: forest green silk bottom with nude lace top and so on.

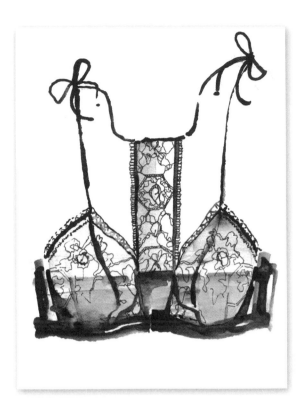

Confidence begins at the innermost layer, and so does clothing confidence. The first thing you put on your body when you get out of the shower is equally as important as the last accessory you add before you walk out the door. "Why, Dallas? No one will see it!" *You* will, and that will change how you feel about yourself. I bet you'll walk faster, stand taller, and maybe even smile when you order your morning skinny vanilla latte.

Hours before the Victoria's Secret fashion show last year, I was sitting backstage with the models and I asked one, "Do you really feel confi-

✳ Get measured by a professional. It's free, and don't you dare think twice about questioning your size. Listen to the lady with the measuring tape.

dent as you walk or are you nervous?" She replied, "Have you seen what I get to wear in the show? How could I not feel sexy in it?"

Does a little lace underneath your clothes give you the extra confidence you'll need throughout the day? Let's find out.

This prep week, wear your nicest set of delicates. Lay the set out before you hop in the shower, and after you get out, put on some moisturizer, the set, and then whatever clothes you had planned on—whether it's your work clothes or lounge clothes.

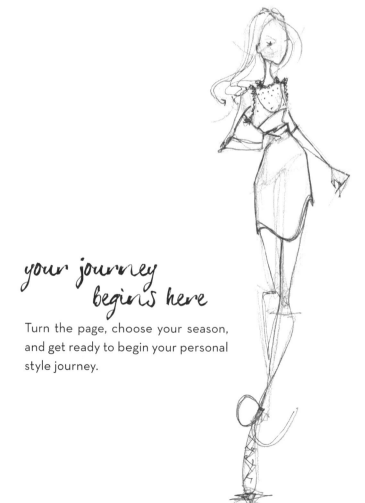

your journey begins here

Turn the page, choose your season, and get ready to begin your personal style journey.

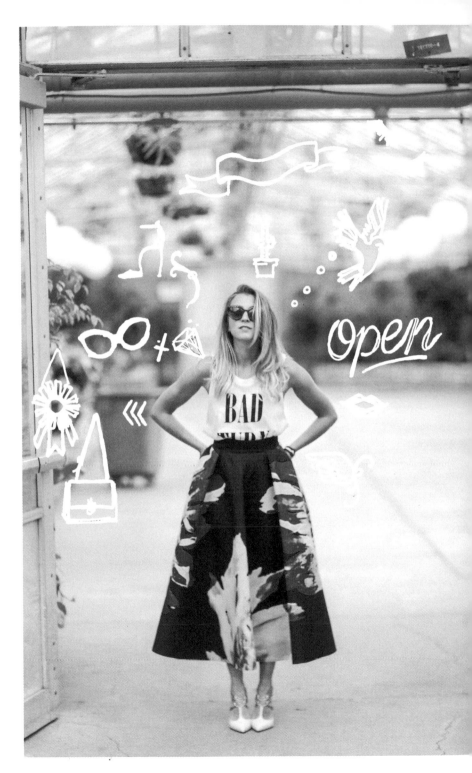

SPRING

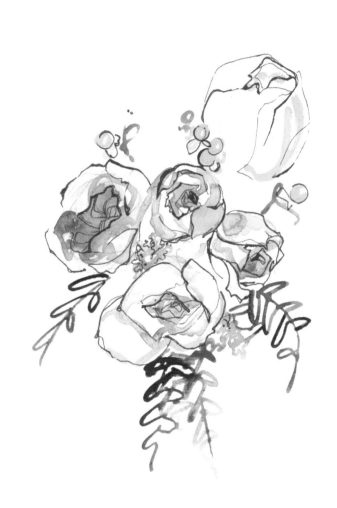

The season of fresh flowers and fresh starts, spring is the perfect time to begin a journey of self-renewal. Coral lips and pink pedicures begin to replace the deep, intense shades of winter. Store windows fill up with feminine pastel palettes. There are cherry blossoms blooming, birds chirping and butterflies in the air. Spring = pure romance. It was designed for dinners outside and open-back dresses.

After I'm done twirling through the park rejoicing that the sun is actually still a thing, I get started on my spring ensemble strategy. (Which mostly involves packing up about 187 wool sweaters and outerwear excess, and then lugging them into storage.) After I stow away all my winter gear, I bring in the soft, flowy pieces that make up my spring uniform.

Everything gets a little bit lighter. Spirits, denim shades, my wallet.

I'm ready to wear floral as far as the eye can see, and stripes will become my everyday staple. I find myself making time for daily walks and sleeping with the windows open in the evening. I might even start that workout schedule that never happened in January.

The smell of fresh-cut grass makes me want to kick off my shoes and run in it.

The hiiiills are aliiiive . . .

Throw open your windows and take inspiration from your garden.

Your spring goal? Embrace the season along with its shorter hemlines. Don't switch over to summer mode just yet—stop and smell the roses.

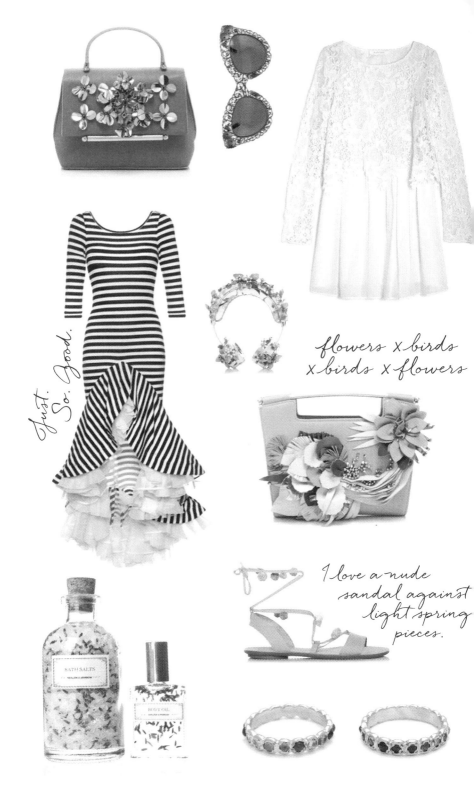

flowers x birds x birds x flowers

Just. So. Good.

I love a nude sandal against light spring pieces.

BATH SALTS

BODY OIL

#thingsweneed

I'll take
two, k
thanks.

mix prints flawlessly

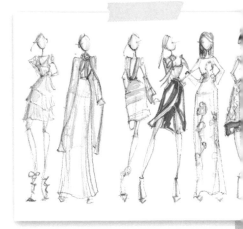

Every It girl has mastered one very important fashion statement: pattern play. She waltzes into a casual lunch in her printed culottes and loose patterned shirt, and you think, *How does that outfit even work together?* But it does! While fashion girls are generally comfortable with print mixing, it scares the heck out of just about everyone else. Let's break it down.

There is one formula for flawlessly mixing prints. Follow it to match up to four items, and become a mix master.

Top + shoes = match (in color or pattern)
bottoms + accessories = same undertones

Voilà! Mix master.

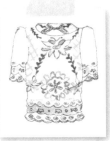

✱ All mixed up and feeling like it, too? Add a solid accessory to ground your look.

EASE IN

- Incorporate a print into an otherwise solid outfit and make the second print an accessory that you won't always have on—maybe a jacket or a bag. By the end of the day you'll feel more comfortab[le] with the overall idea and will be ready for your next step.
- Try inverse colors. Wear a black garment with white accents and [a] white garment with black accents.

STEP IT UP

- Wear a print and a solid piece that complement each other. Then switch the solid for a pattern in the same shade for two prints that "just work."

  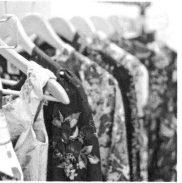

  - Pair up base colors. If you have an item of clothing that is mostly one color, pair it with another item that is mostly one color.

  ✳ Still too shy to get started? Start off by wearing a print with a classic chambray shirt (you know, the denim-y shirts that aren't a heavy denim). Take the look straight from work to dinner, and soon enough, you'll be ready to take your pattern play to the next level.

SCALE IS IMPORTANT. Large prints pair well with small prints, and vice versa. (Wide stripes with smaller flowers and narrow stripes with bigger flowers.)

COLOR FAMILY MATTERS. Match colors, not prints. Look for prints with the same undertones.

DON'T GO OVERBOARD. The goal is to look effortless, not busy.

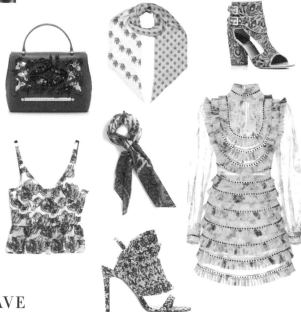

FEELING BRAVE

- After you've mastered wearing two prints, add a third. Make it a neutral pattern with similar undertones.
- Try a printed scarf over a printed top or romper. Now you're a print mixer and a layering expert all in one.

reflect }

well, aren't you ms. fancy pants

Nothing gives a breezier feeling than a casual girl in a printed pant. Today, be that girl. Hit the dressing room with a small pattern that will hardly feel like a print at all for your most flattering option. Here are ways to try this lighthearted and relaxed look.

Don't feel overwhelmed at the large selection of prints in stores. Choose one you think is pretty and don't overanalyze it.

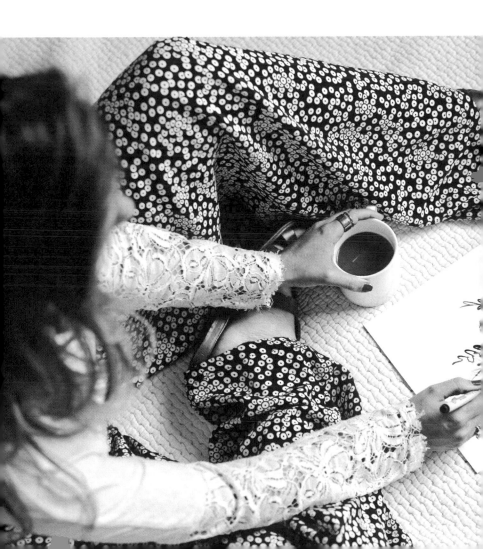

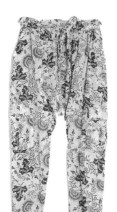

EASE IN

- Cropped ankle pants, with a lightweight cashmere sweater, nude leather sandal, and a killer tan.

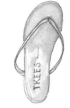

- Loose-fitted printed pants give an easygoing vibe, while a fitted style can look classic. Play around and see what suits your personality best. (I'm loose and laid back 95 percent of the time.)

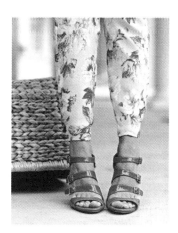

FEELING BRAVE

A wide-leg high-waisted pair in a silky fabric. Belt this and it looks just like a maxi skirt.

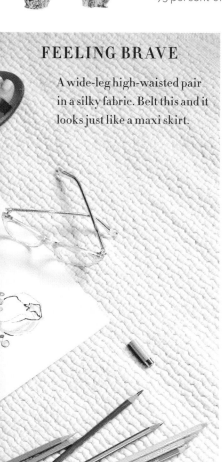

STEP IT UP

- Slouchy pants with a jogger leg and pockets, a V-neck tee, and a flat slide or sandal.

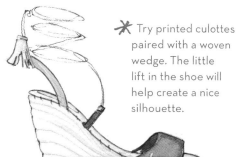

- Try printed culottes paired with a woven wedge. The little lift in the shoe will help create a nice silhouette.

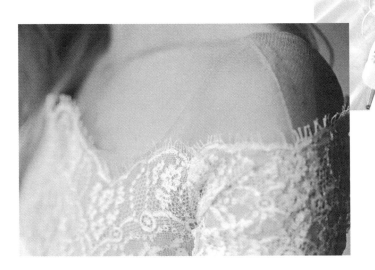

✳ Shop in unexpected places. Bridal stores carry not only lace heels and booties, but the most beautiful lace tops I've ever seen. My favorite: Bhldn.

get laced

Chantilly. Alençon. Guipure. There isn't a single lace style that I don't love. Lace is one of my biggest inspirations. I dare you to sit at a Marchesa or Reem Acra show and not become equally obsessed. While I wear touches of lace throughout all seasons, most of my lace pieces live within my spring wardrobe because the weather is ideal for the wear. This challenge isn't about looking like a bridesmaid; it's a reminder that a little lace touch can give a feminine, delicate feel to your look.

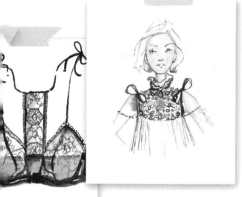

EASE IN

- Keep a delicate lace robe hanging on the back of your door and wear it during your morning routine.
- Wear a lace silk cami underneath it all. (I wear these year-round under all my sweaters instead of those stretchy too-tight tanks.)
- New pastel-colored lace undies for the season are always a good idea.

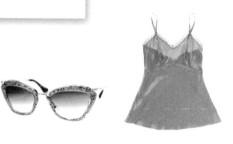

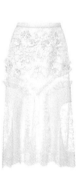

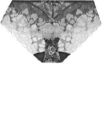

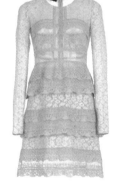

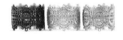

TEP IT UP

Try long lacy sleeves (I especially love this paired with something straw).

A lace babydoll dress with a gladiator sandal.

Black lace heels paired with a black silk jumpsuit (or pants) and a lariat necklace.

FEELING BRAVE

- A lace pencil skirt with a T-shirt, a nude heel, and shades.
- Silky shorts trimmed in lace, paired with a sweatshirt and flats.
- A lace dress in a bright color, with nude shoes and a clutch. Feels. So. Classic.

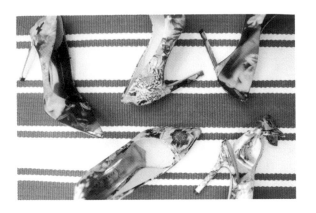

perfect pairings
we go together like:

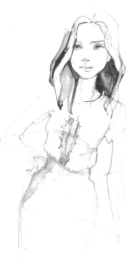

{ *stripes* × *floral* }
The best of the mixed prints.
A striped top with a floral skirt
and open-toed T-straps is my
favorite combination.

graphic tees
× *pencil skirts*
I like mine with rolled sleeves, shades, a clutch, and
heels.

Graphic tee feeling too young for you? You can
try this with a solid tee, too.

spring skirts
× *winter sweaters*
On a breezy night, bring along a heavy winter sweater and
throw it over a spring dress or a light airy skirt for a fun
combo. I like mine with a light-colored cross-body bag.

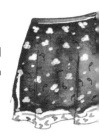

Therapy Check-in

hey lady,

Time for a little self-love.

Take some time to ask yourself how all these challenges are going. By now you're probably seeing some interesting changes, not only in your wardrobe but in yourself.

1. WHAT'S ONE WORD THAT DESCRIBES YOUR PERSONAL STYLE TODAY?

2. DOES WHAT YOU'RE WEARING TODAY MAKE YOU FEEL GOOD?

3. WHAT'S ONE THING YOU ARE BEGINNING TO UNDERSTAND ABOUT YOUR PERSONAL STYLE?

4. WHAT ARE YOU ENJOYING LEARNING ABOUT YOURSELF DURING THIS PROCESS?

5. WHAT DO YOU NEED TO TAKE MORE TIME FOR IN ORDER TO LIVE YOUR MOST STYLISH LIFE?

6. ARE YOU TAKING THE TIME YOU PROMISED YOURSELF?

7. ARE YOU TAKING TIME TO ENJOY THE BEAUTIFUL THINGS AROUND YOU?

Confetti!!

I'm proud of your dedication (*and honesty*).

Your journey is just beginning. Now go and do something nice for yourself. I think you deserve it. How will you reward yourself?

Design Your
Spring Palette

Bye-bye navy, emerald, and crimson. See you in a few months. For the spring, I long for rich rosy pinks inspired by cotton-candy skies. I add wispy violets, mint, and very light, silvery blues to the clothing rack. Just when my closet is starting to look like a straight-up Easter egg, I change lanes, adding neutrals and a few small additions of brights *(a coral here, a poppy There)*. Building my spring wardrobe is just like mixing colors for me, and this palette is a dream.

Everything feels cheerier in springtime, and so should your wardrobe. Let's design your spring color palette.

It's time to create your own spring color story. Place your notes or inspiration here:

what colors haven't you worn before

which colors you would be open to trying

the color you wear most often in the spring

did you just say black? I can't with you.

how that color makes you feel

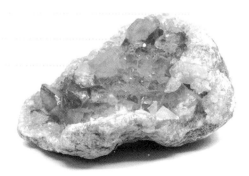

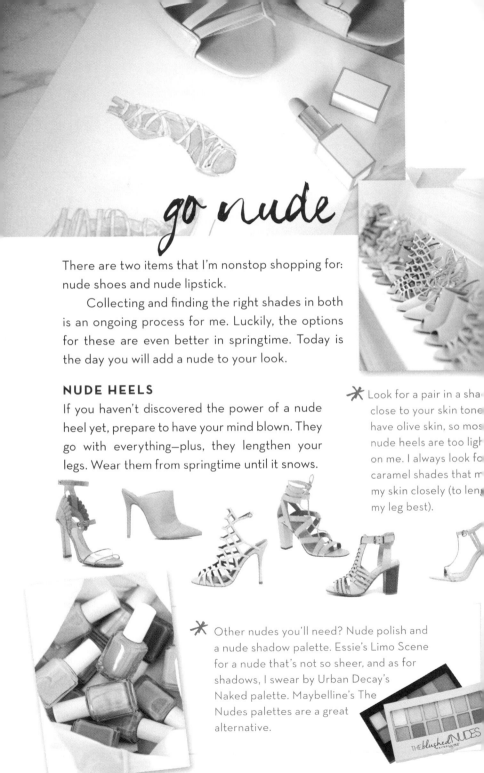

go nude

There are two items that I'm nonstop shopping for: nude shoes and nude lipstick.

Collecting and finding the right shades in both is an ongoing process for me. Luckily, the options for these are even better in springtime. Today is the day you will add a nude to your look.

NUDE HEELS

If you haven't discovered the power of a nude heel yet, prepare to have your mind blown. They go with everything—plus, they lengthen your legs. Wear them from springtime until it snows.

✳ Look for a pair in a sha[de] close to your skin tone[. I] have olive skin, so mos[t] nude heels are too lig[ht] on me. I always look fo[r] caramel shades that m[atch] my skin closely (to len[gthen] my leg best).

✳ Other nudes you'll need? Nude polish and a nude shadow palette. Essie's Limo Scene for a nude that's not so sheer, and as for shadows, I swear by Urban Decay's Naked palette. Maybelline's The Nudes palettes are a great alternative.

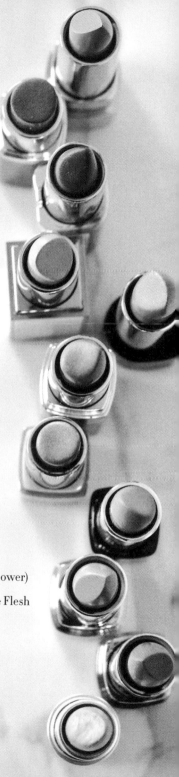

NUDE LIPSTICK

Try. This. On. You're looking for something that enhances your natural lip color, so look for a hue one shade darker than the natural color of your lip. Grab a liner in a nude as well so you don't lose volume.

Nude lipsticks look different on everyone. One lip shade can look completely different from person to person because of the natural base color of your lip. When trying shades on, make sure the color isn't too chalky.

the twelve nude lippys you can't live without:

And the winners are:

- Dolce & Gabbana Classic Cream lipstick in Honey
- bareMinerals Marvelous Moxie lipstick in Soft Nude
- Estée Lauder Pure Color Envy in Naked Ambition
- Tata Harper Volumizing Lip and Cheek Tint in Very Vivacious (I keep backups of this)
- Lancôme L'Absolu Rouge in Jeweled Pink
- Yves Saint Laurent Vernis À Lèvres Glossy Stain in Corail Mutin (that's fancy for "peachy coral")
- Stila Stay All Day in Dolce or Patina (for serious staying power)
- Make Up For Ever Rouge Artist Intense Lipstick in Matte Flesh
- Tarte Tarteist Creamy Matte Lip Paint in tbt mauve
- NARS Lipstick in Bilbao
- L'Oréal Colour Riche Lipcolour in Fairest Nude
- Lipstick Queen Saint Lipstick in Pinky Nude

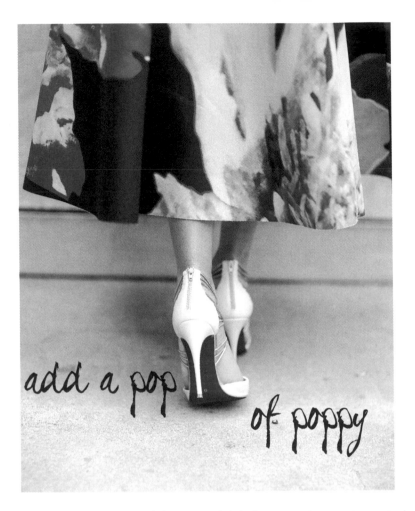

add a pop of poppy

Christian Louboutin's red bottoms didn't become the most coveted soles in fashion by accident. Those dashes of red on the bottoms of every fashionista's foot racing across Fifth Avenue grabbed attention for one good reason.

{ red } *The color of passion*

Some won't wear it because they feel it draws *too* much attention, but I'm willing to bet this next challenge will make you feel like a siren. I vote for wearing just a touch (a lip color or nail polish when nothing else in the look is red) or going all in (a red dress with a deep red coat in the winter).

Three unexpected occasions to try a red lip:

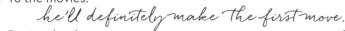

1. On vacation. *she must be parisian.*
2. To the movies.
   he'll definitely make the first move.
3. During the day.
   your groceries just got so glam.

EASE IN

⚹ Start with one small touch:
a shoe, your nails, or a bold red lip.

STEP IT UP

⚹ Pair a bright red with shades of white, camel,
and pinks. Use this page as your color guide.

FEELING BRAVE

⚹ Add some sparkle or maybe an
unexpected color, like teal or
green, to your look.

deborah lippmann

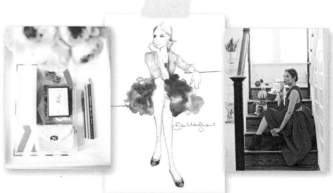

{ *reflect* }

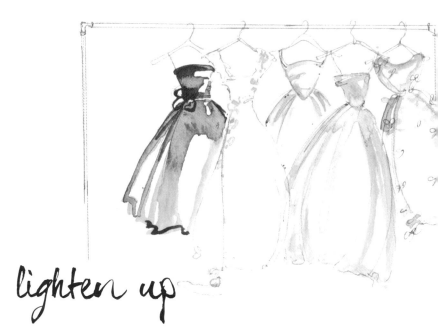

lighten up

Self-proclaimed pastel-phobe? Too bad. Been told pastels don't work for your coloring? Bust that myth! This challenge is to incorporate some soft, whisper-light hues into your ensemble. Our goal? To prove once and for all that pastels aren't just for Easter eggs. They're for everyone!

Start by choosing a few key items of your look (tops/bottoms) in a soft neutral like white, cream, camel, or gray and build the rest of your outfit from there.

»———→ MINI CHALLENGE ←———«

Try this palette with fresh waves. Loose, pretty hair complements the gentle tones.

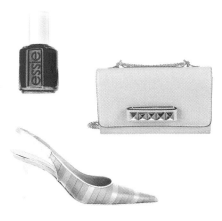

EASE IN

- Try a pastel accessory, like a clutch or a purse, with a bright red polish.
- A sweet pastel nail color paired with leather strappy sandals.

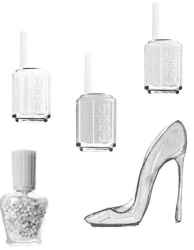

STEP IT UP

- Color block two pastels, like a pink skirt with a peach top, or a light lemony sweater with violet flats.
- Stack multiples of pastel jewelry (bracelets or necklaces) for an unexpected addition.

FEELING BRAVE

- Mix two or three pastel colors, add a gray into the mix and a bright lip.
- Pair a mix of sugary pastels with a dash of a deep color, like oxblood, to ground the mix.

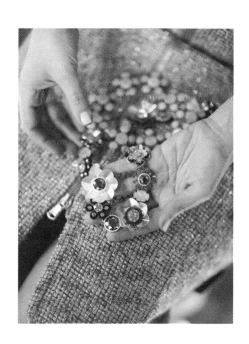

FOUR MUST-HAVE PASTEL PIECES FOR SPRING

1. blazer
2. bag
3. dress
4. silk camisole

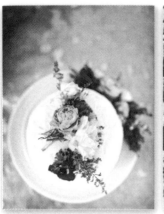
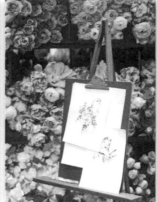
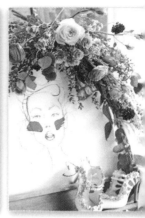

EASE IN

- A floral shirtdress and wedges.
- A loose-fitting floral top with white denim shorts and dark aviators.
- A floral print on your purse.

STEP IT UP

- Sleeveless floral maxi with strappy sandals and thin hoops.
- A floral kimono over a fluttery white dress.
- Pair a floral romper with flat gladiator sandals for the beach.

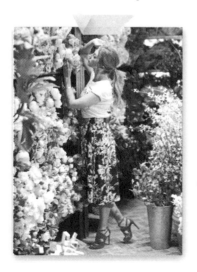

FEELING BRAVE

- Floral pants with a mule and a sheer mani.
- A lacy floral skirt with a gray T-shirt and sandals.
- A long-sleeved floral-print dress with a shimmery gloss.

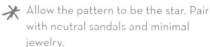
Allow the pattern to be the star. Pair with neutral sandals and minimal jewelry.

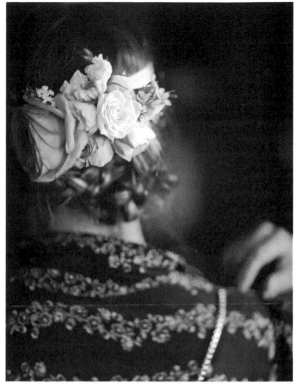

✳ Look for bouquets in watercolor prints and with bold, bright groupings that suit your taste.

freshen up with floral

Whether you are the girl who has four floral-print shirts in her closet and always has her eye open for lucky number five, or the girl who stays away from the unapologetically feminine print, florals are always in style in spring. Wear a floral print today, and I guarantee you'll feel a little more romantic than usual.

≫—→ MINI CHALLENGE ←—≪

buy yourself fresh flowers. just for you. just because.

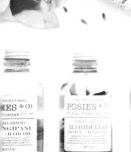

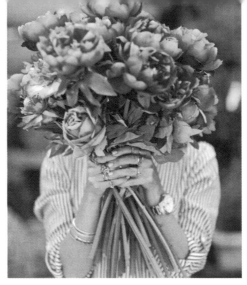

Stop and smell the r

everything's coming up rose-y

Add a little rose to your routine. Come on, it's spring!

A few years ago I started picking up fresh roses for myself each week. The weekly treat then grew to fresh roses and a splash of rosewater. Then, fresh roses and rosewater and fragrance, and my obsession turned into addiction. The flower, the color, the scent, the metal... Roses soon took over my workspace and social channels alike. Take a cue from every mood board in our office and start seeing the world through our rose-tinted glasses. Here is some inspiration on where to begin.

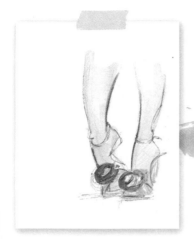

Take a few minutes to journal about how well you are doing with your challenges.

{ reflect }

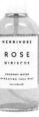
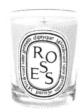
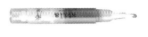

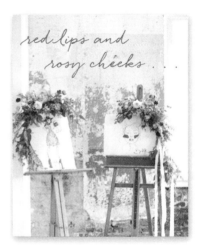

red lips and rosy cheeks . . .

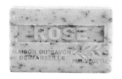
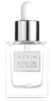

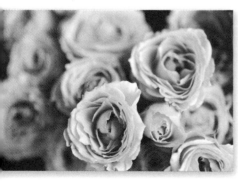

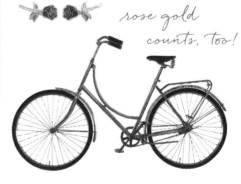

rose gold counts, too!

*he loves me,
he loves me not,
he loves me . . .*

get more wear out of your essential striped shirt

Plain white tee feeling a little meh?
Bring in the stripes!
  Stripes are the "neutral" print of the world, and this spring, you'll need to get more wear out of your go-to striped shirt. The possibilities are endless with this wardrobe workhorse, so if you don't have one, it's time to get one. A loose-fitted tee with a thin stripe or a button-down classic—the impact is the same. Choose one you like and try to bring it to the front of the closet more often.

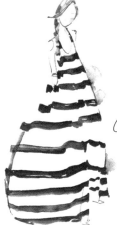

»»→ MINI CHALLENGE ←««

Add a simple, comfy, striped dress to your wardrobe and get ready to live in it.

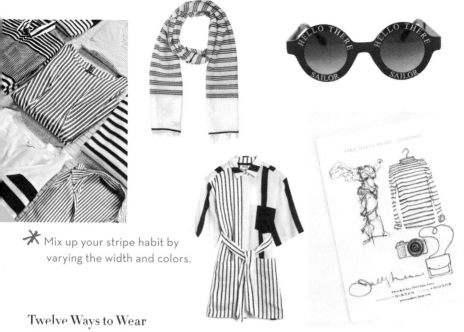

✳ Mix up your stripe habit by
varying the width and colors.

Twelve Ways to Wear
the Essential Striped Shirt:

1. With a midi skirt and booties.
2. With a print. Basically any print, and florals, obvi (see Perfect Pairings, page 48).
3. With a classic trench coat and a '70s-inspired chunky heel.
4. Blouse-y and buttoned with a loose paisley silk scarf.
5. With cropped white pants, espadrille flats, a pony, and aviators.
6. With a fancier black skirt and a clutch, for an evening out.
7. Under a black leather jacket (see the leather jacket challenge, page 154) with undone hair.
8. With dark denim, black heels, a dark clutch, and a single bracelet.
9. With denim shorts, leather flat sandals, and piles of beaded and woven bracelets.
10. A turtleneck worn with high-waisted pants and a denim jacket.
11. A button-down with denim shorts, sandals, and a leather strap watch or designer belt.
12. A striped dress with an overcoat over your shoulders, heels, and a bag tucked under your arm.

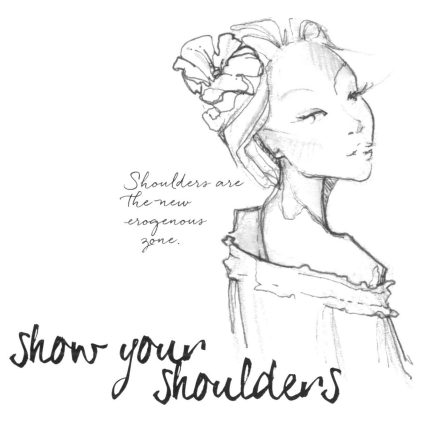

Shoulders are the new erogenous zone.

show your shoulders

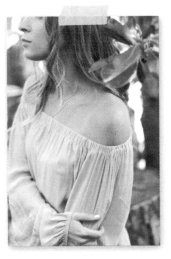

When the weather is a little warmer, but not warm enough for me to change over my entire closet to its official sunshine state, a shoulder-skimming top is a nice solution.

EASE IN

- Keep it simple with white jeans and leather sandals.

✳ Still too shy to get started? Shoulder cutouts have the same effect. Try this look for date night.

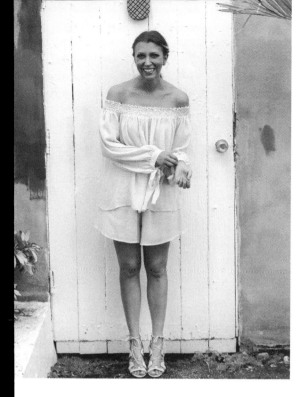

STEP IT UP

⚞ If you feel too bare, just add heels and a delicate necklace or drop earrings. (The cut of this blouse will highlight what sits above it. Choose your jewelry accordingly.)

FEELING BRAVE

⚞ An off-the-shoulder dress is a flirty option and will take you right into summer.

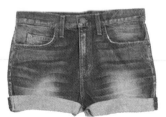

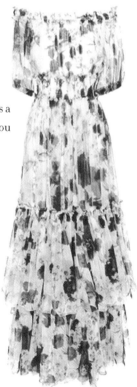

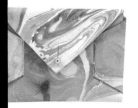

how i wear mine:
With a clutch, a loose bun, and a pair of boyfriend shorts.

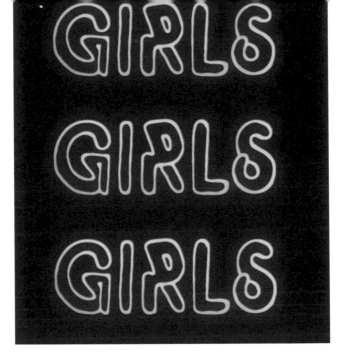

flirty and feminine

Maybe it's because my legs haven't seen the sun in months that I want to show them off as much as possible once the temperature rises. Forget about short or tight skirts for this challenge and instead turn to midi and maxi skirts with fuller shapes to enhance your figure. What's wrong with getting a little flirty? Get out your dresses, skirts, and feminine silhouettes, and get ready to turn heads.

Psst: skirts just not your thing?
fine. a high-waisted pant with a delicately
ruffled top works, too. tuck it in.
i want to see your curves today!

EASE IN

- Try a midi skirt and a chambray shirt. Tie it in the front to show off that skirt shape even more.
- An A-line knee-length skirt with a cuffed-sleeve button-down and heels. Pair with a casual pony and minimal makeup to play off the polished skirt.

STEP IT UP

- A pencil skirt with a T-shirt, heels, and a bright bag. Sleek shades look nice here, too.
- Get extra girly and add something with a bow detail. A polished version of your pointed-toe flats makes the look without looking juvenile.

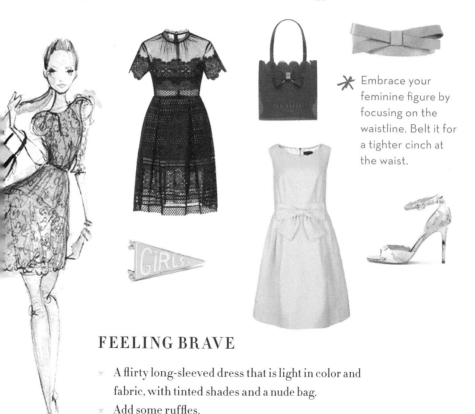

✳ Embrace your feminine figure by focusing on the waistline. Belt it for a tighter cinch at the waist.

FEELING BRAVE

- A flirty long-sleeved dress that is light in color and fabric, with tinted shades and a nude bag.
- Add some ruffles.

✳ Legs not in summer shape yet? An airbrush spray or spray tan will help mask ghostly winter skin.

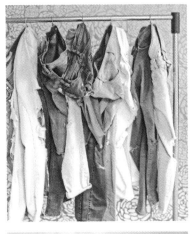
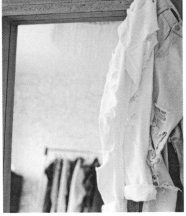
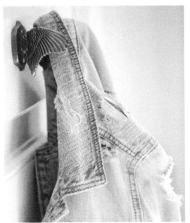
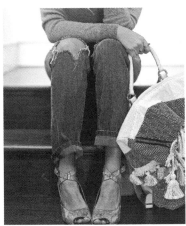

get ripped

Every single time I walk into my grandfather's suit shop with ripped denim, he makes the same exact joke: "I hope you didn't pay for those. They are ripped." Unfortunately, yes, Gramp—I paid a pretty penny for these. Whether you're showing a little knee or half your leg, ripped denim is a staple of today's times. All those splits make your jeans-and-tee uniform feel even more relaxed.

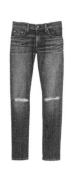
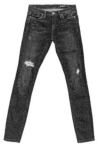

EASE IN

- Try a pair with a small rip at the knee, a jacket, and shades.
- Mix 'em up with a preppy top.
- Roll the bottoms just an inch, and add nude heels and a statement earring.

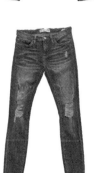

* Pay attention to size. They're not giving you a relaxed feel if they're stopping the circulation to your legs. On the other side, if they're too loose, they will make you look much larger than you actually are. Try these on to get them just right.

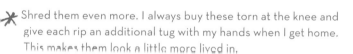

* Shred them even more. I always buy these torn at the knee and give each rip an additional tug with my hands when I get home. This makes them look a little more lived in.

STEP IT UP

- With a lace or embellished top and a black bag with piles of gold jewelry.
- Topped with a sweater that is soft in color or style and patent loafers.
- Juxtapose the tears above with a pair of sleek boots.

FEELING BRAVE

- With a trench coat, a cross-body bag, and chunky sandals.
- A cropped embellished jacket and a skinny belt.
- With a denim top, simple black ankle-strap heels, and a nude lip.

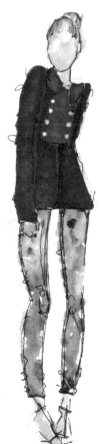

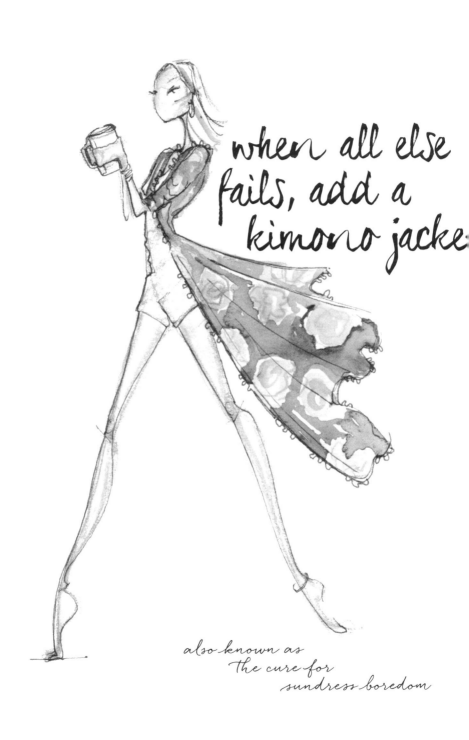

when all else fails, add a kimono jacket

also known as
the cure for
sundress boredom

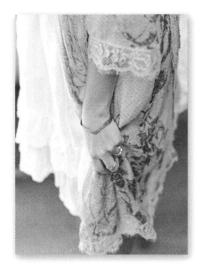

No, not that kind. I know you're picturing the traditional Japanese garment, but I'm talking about the very gypsy-like, light and airy version of a cardigan. Sometimes in the summer we need that something special, but it's hot, so extra layers are unthinkable. Enter the kimono to solve all your basic jean short and T-shirt problems.

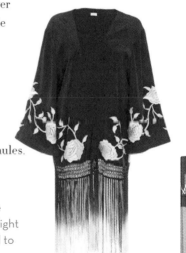

EASE IN

- Floral sheer kimonos with brushed silver jewelry and a dash of lip gloss add a little drifter spirit to your day.
- Belted and paired with a choker.

STEP IT UP

- With a romper and booties.
- Over a tucked-in silk shirt with black mules.

✳ A kimono jacket makes an excellent choice for traveling. It's comfy on the plane, and you always have an extra light layer with you if you get cold or need to update your look while on the road.

FEELING BRAVE

- Throw it on over a maxi dress for an instant update.
- Wear one belted without a top underneath to create a deep V.

wanderer . . .

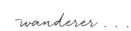

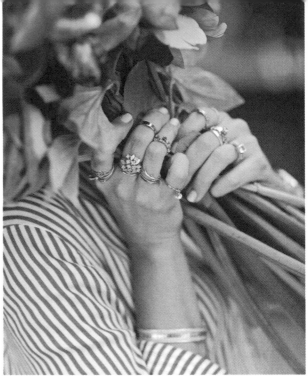

mix your metals

This year I worked on a design collaboration with Dawes Design, and I asked my social following to weigh in on the ring color. I heard about one million "rules," including:

> "Choose silver so it goes with everything."
> "I wouldn't choose gold because it only matches with my antique jewelry."
> "Rose gold doesn't complement anything."

The need for this challenge was clear.

I don't care how you do it: rose gold and silver, gold and rose gold, gold, silver and rose gold together . . . but mix them up and make them the focus of your look.

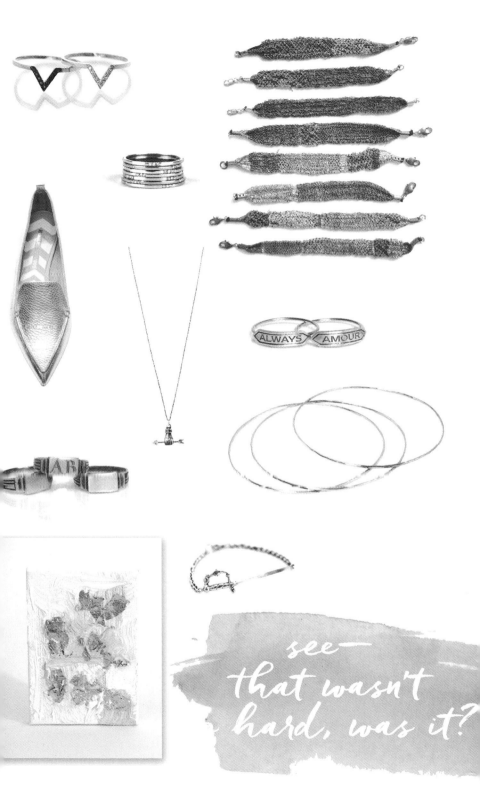

see—
that wasn't
hard, was it?

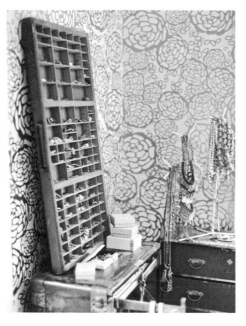

As a jewelry collector and sometimes jewelry designer, I have an extensive jewelry collection that I am very attached to. I collect pieces during my trips and travels, and each piece feels like a little part of me. I'd rather wear a tiny delicate star wrapped around my pinky that reminds me of moonlit nights in Vienna than bring home twenty tchotchkes. My jewelry collection is full of little moments from my life, and I personally don't like it tucked away in boxes.

It's one thing to collect jewelry; it's another thing altogether to display it. Whether your collection is small or large, I believe that displaying your most-loved pieces gives you a sense of joy when you see them each morning.

put your jewelry on display

Plus, it reminds you to wear your treasures more often. Let's design your personal jewelry storage solutions. Here are some of mine as a guide:

MY PERSONAL JEWELRY STORAGE SOLUTIONS

Lined in pink velvet, I keep **vintage jewelry boxes** open so I can see the trinkets and the velvet inside. *swoooon*

I keep my earrings in a **letterpress drawer** that I have leaning up against the wall. The individual wooden rectangles act as a proud showcase to highlight each special pair.

My thick statement necklaces hang on a sturdy **necklace stand,** and my thin ones hang from a stand of stacked branches. Hanging thin neck-

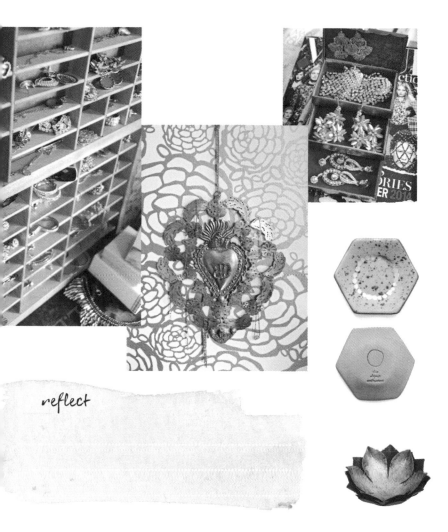

reflect

laces neatly gives a polished look and keeps the chains from tangling.

Chunky bracelets get laid neatly in a **glass box**. The trickiest pieces to find a place for were my thin bracelets. Look for unexpected places to hang these together. I chose an antique silver Milagros heart.

While some of my rings go in the letterpress box, I also keep a few beautiful ceramic ring dishes sprinkled around the space. I've seen people use tiered cake stands for large pieces as well.

as you look at your collection on display, how do you feel?

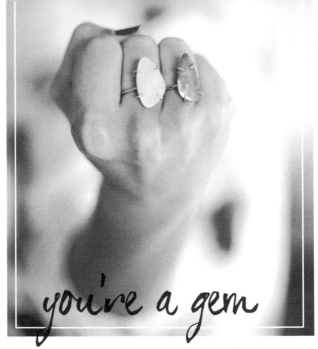

you're a gem

*it's time to admit something.
i have an infatuation with opal.*

I've always been drawn to opal. It was only later in life, after I built my opal collection, that I found out the stone is said to aid in visualization, imagination, and dreams. And it's not a bit surprising to me that opal is associated with emotions. There seems to be an entire dreamy sunset and/or sunny ocean scene within each stone. That minty teal shade with tiny flecks of yellow and pink... *it gives me all of the feels*.

I wasn't born in October, so I'm living proof that you don't have to pick your birthstone when choosing your gem. Go by your gut reaction to the stone and the color.

HOW TO CHOOSE YOUR PERFECT ROCK

AMETHYST—*healing* x *protection*

AMBER—*divine* x *positivity*

DIAMOND—*purity* x *consciousness*

HEMATITE—*grounding* x *clarity*

LAPIS—*wisdom* x *intuition*

MOONSTONE—*balance* x *femininity*

OPAL—*creativity* x *imagination*

PEARL—*heart* x *stress reduction*

QUARTZ—*energy* x *healing*

ROSE QUARTZ—*harmony* x *balance*

TURQUOISE—*love* x *spiritual*

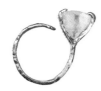

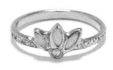

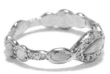

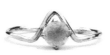

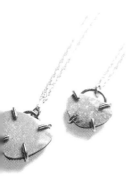

Think about:
- which gemstone color you're drawn to and why
- which meaning you relate to the most
- which would you choose as your personal gemstone?

That's that. Let the jewelry search begin.
I choose .... as my personal gemstone.

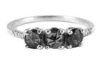
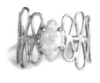

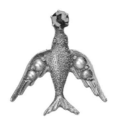
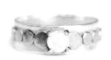
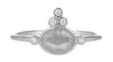

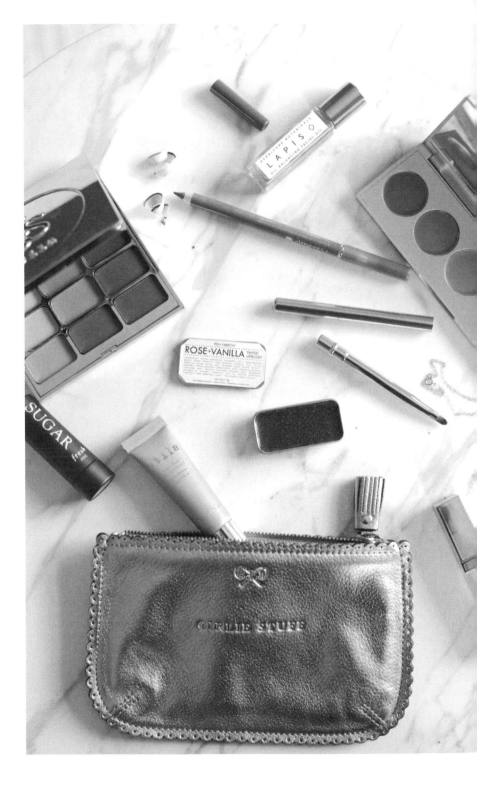

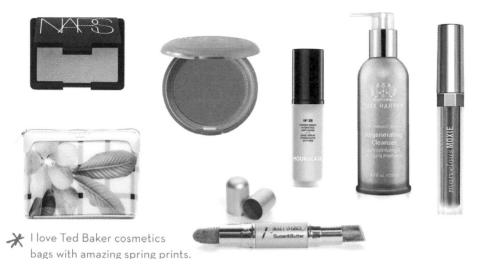

✳ I love Ted Baker cosmetics
bags with amazing spring prints.

I often say if I wasn't a fashion illustrator I'd be a makeup artist. I have a very steady hand and laugh in the face of liquid eyeliner (even the most challenging tip won't ruin my confidence). I look forward to a change of season because for me that means a change of my color palette. For spring, switch over to lightweight creams, fresh scents, and bright shades. Color has an effect on you visually so get ready for your mood to lift with every a.m. application.

freshen up your spring makeup bag

#THINGSWENEED

Lightweight foundation	Lip tints
Rosy cheeks	
Floral scents	
Highlighter pencils	
Glossy pastel polish	

rock a bright lip

The fun thing about a bright lip is that any of
the shades on page 81 look perfect paired with the following
makeup. Master this simple palette on your face and then switch
your bright lips as you wish.

#THINGSWENEED

Foundation	Eye shadow	Blush
Bronzer	Eye liner	Bright lip shade of
Setting powder	Mascara	your choice

1. Start with a fresh complexion, a foundation, and a bronzer, then use a setting powder to get a nice matte finish.
2. Add shimmery golden brown eye shadow and a touch of thin ink liner across your top lid only.
3. Black lengthening mascara and a nice pinky-brown blush (just for depth here, no additional pops of color needed) will complete the look.
4. Simply add your bright lip choice for a classic spring look.

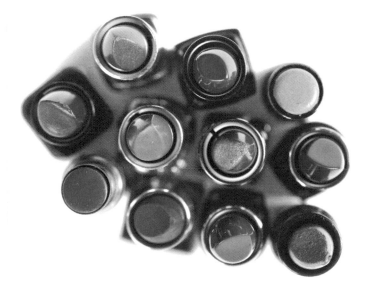

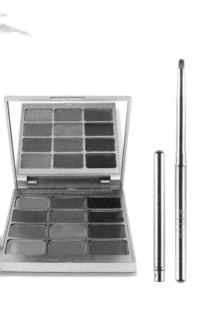

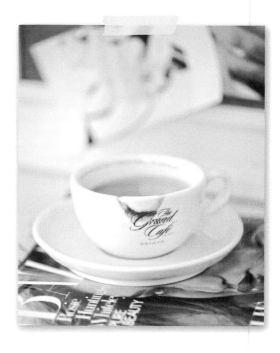

{ reflect }

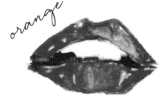

orange

....

....

....

SHADES TO TRY }

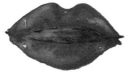

bright
pink

berry

coral

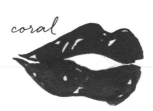

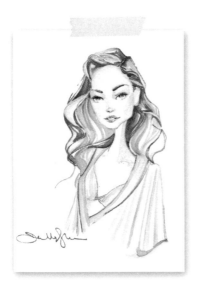

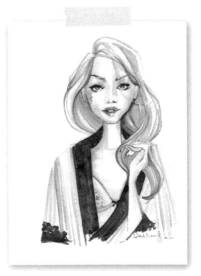

get beach waves

Some days it's not about the clothes. It's about the hair and the shoes. (Actually, it's always about the shoes—wait until you get to Winter, page 193.) And on those days you want to go for bombshell waves.

GET TOUSLED TRESSES
IN SIX EASY STEPS

1. Spray completely dry hair with dry shampoo for lots of volume.
2. Using a clip-less curling iron (or my personal favorite, the Beachwaver), separate your hair into 1-inch sections as you go. Always curl away from your face and never curl the ends (this is the key to the perfectly imperfect wave).
3. Once all your hair is curled, pin up a few curls around your face with hairpins to set those pieces.

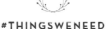

#THINGSWENEED

Curling iron
Dry shampoo
Wax spray

4. After a few minutes, remove the pins. Flip your head over and lightly separate the curls with your fingers.
5. Flip your hair back and see how the curls fall.
6. Spray all over generously with a wax spray to hold. Place your fingers on your scalp and massage the product in to get that perfect rumpled bedhead look.

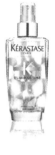 Continue to add dry shampoo throughout the day for volume and touch-ups.

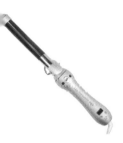
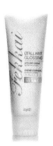
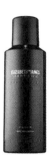
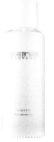

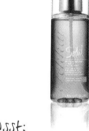

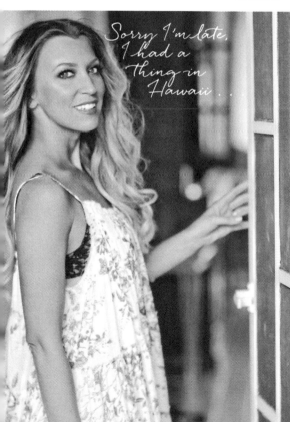

Sorry I'm late, I had a thing in Hawaii...

Psst:
Don't have time today? Grab a sea salt spray.

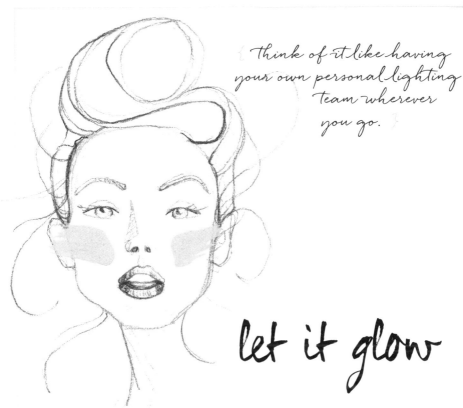

Think of it like having your own personal lighting team wherever you go.

let it glow

Highlighter. It's the secret weapon in every makeup artist's bag. Years ago, one such artist told me that the single thing you should add to your beauty routine every day is a good highlighter. It makes you feel better, look healthier, and simply be more radiant. I never thought I could be that bright-skinned girl, but he made me vow to try to make this a habit, so I took on his challenge: to use highlighter, not here and there, but daily. This changed my look so much that I am passing it on not so much as a challenge, but a mantra.

WHAT TO LOOK FOR IN A HIGHLIGHTER AND BRUSH

Highlighter should shimmer, not glitter. It will look like a pressed powder with a twinkle in it.

Make sure the brush has delicate bristles (to avoid stripes). I like a fan brush for this.

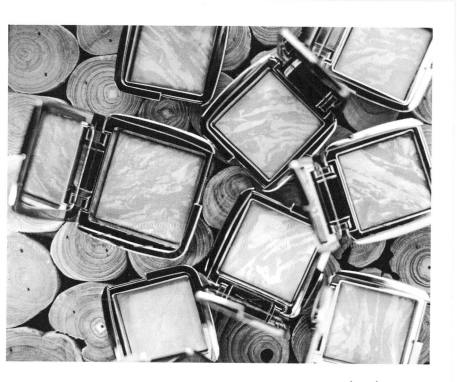

1. Quickly, without much thought and with a good amount of product on your brush, swipe in a C shape from the end of your eyebrows to your cheekbones.
2. Then swipe down your nose and hit your chin.
3. The finishing touch is adding a bit to the cupid's bow above your lip. (Oh, hello, Angelina.)

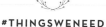

Boom!
Instant radiance.

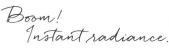

Psst: When I run out of highlighter, a shimmery light eyeshadow will do the trick in a pinch.

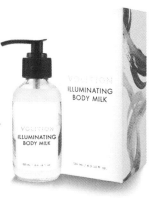

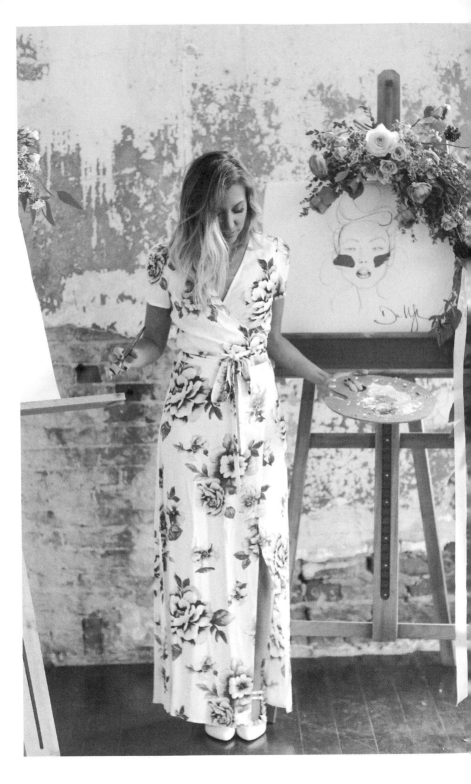

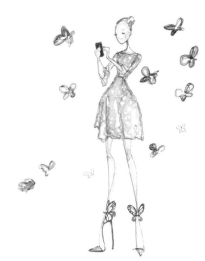

the challenge
continues . . .

PAINT AND PLAY
At the salon this week, choose a nail color you've never worn before. Wearing a new shade can feel adventurous. Defy what conventional color means to you. Teal! Crimson! Nail art? Why not!

KEEP THAT HEALTHY GLOW
This fresh air has us all spending more time outdoors and it's time to step up that exercise regimen. Organize your gym bag, add some fun floral-print activewear today and work out even harder tomorrow. I keep a cute set of workout clothes in my car at all times so I can get out there at a moment's notice.

SPRING CLEANING
Schedule a spring closet-cleaning day and dedicate some time to donate any clothes from the past year that no longer make you feel amazing.

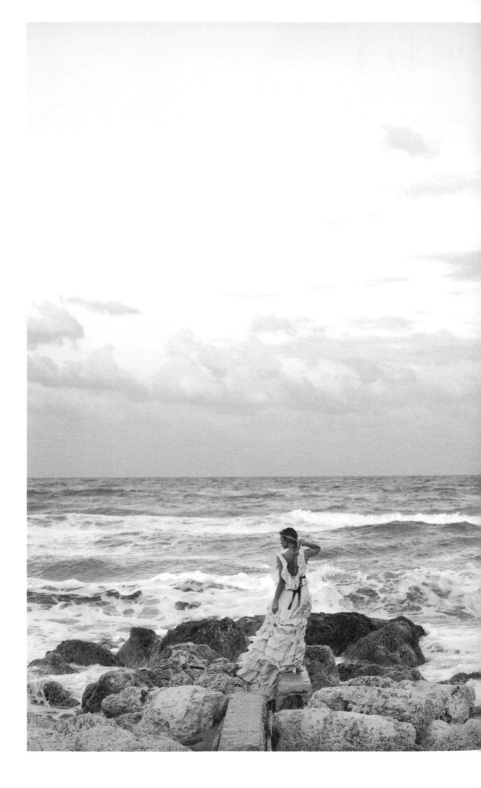

SUMMER

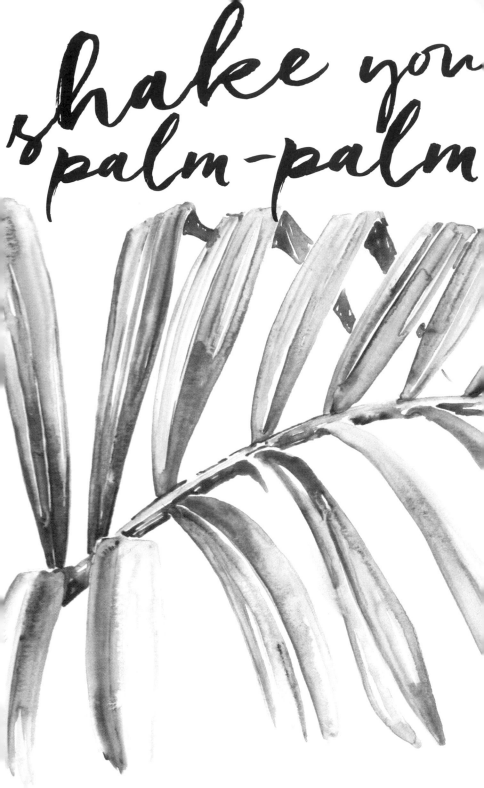

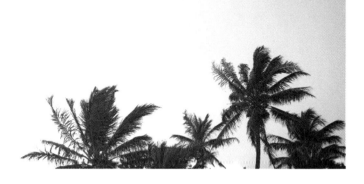

Slip on your sandals and raise your mojitos! Summer is here, and it's time to have a little too much fun in the sun. You don't need a vacation planned to dress like a travel editor all season long. In this section you'll find piles of inspiration on what to wear when the temperature spikes and the invites start pouring in for barbecues, bonfires, and the occasional baseball game.

Breezy V-neck T-shirts in neutrals are my uniform, along with lived-in denim shorts, which also get lighter in color in the summertime. My clothing gets brighter, the fabrics I wear get lighter and looser—even my accessories get smaller and thinner. When I'm on the go in the heat, chasing down a cab, I don't want a single extra thing weighing me down.

Whether you're soaking in the season at the beach, in your own backyard, or in an air-conditioned room at all times, you'll find all the fashion motivation needed to enjoy the nightly fireflies and the sweet scent of funnel cake for as long as possible.

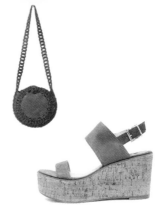

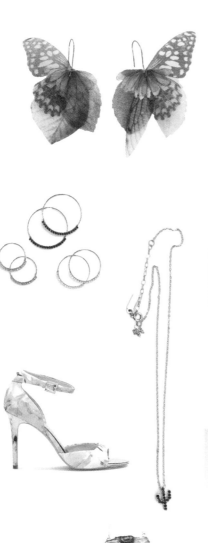

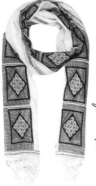

PAINTED DESERT
ROCK SHOP
and cactus farm

Visit the crystal resonance chamber

HIGHWAY 40, SUN VALLEY, AZ

"Don't Blink Or You'll Miss It"

SUCCULENTS AND UNUSUAL CACTI • GEODES • MALACHITE
METEORITE FRAGMENTS • MOON ROCKS • TRILOBITE FOSSILS
TURQUOISE JEWELRY • SALT LAMPS • AMBER • CLOVIS POINTS

RADIO HANDLE: "DESERT FLOWER"

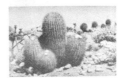

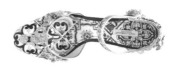

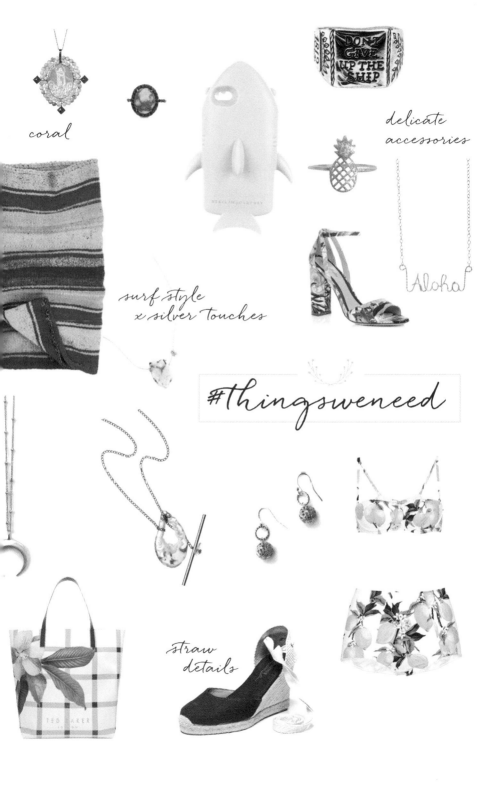

coral

DON'T GIVE UP THE SHIP

delicate accessories

Aloha

surf style x silver touches

#thingsweneed

straw details

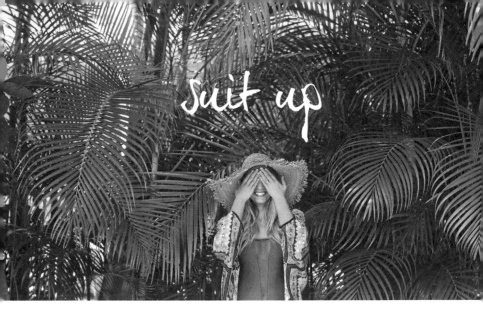

suit up

Ready or not—summer waits for no one. Even though you are likely more excited about the act of going to the beach than you are about wearing a bathing suit in public, by taking the extra time with this challenge to find a swimsuit you feel good in, you'll feel confident by the time you hit the sand. Follow these suggestions and try a group on to see what you feel best in. You can do this in a day at the mall, but don't overlook your favorite online stores. In my humble opinion, the best cuts are most easily found online. Bonus: You can try these on in the comfort of your own home without those horrible fluorescent lights.

Get swimsuit savvy with these suggestions on finding a suit that you love this summer:

Wear a one-piece. A wise woman once told me that the trick to feeling super sexy is to cover up a little. A one-piece is stylish and unexpected, and it's especially nice for active women because you can actually swim and surf comfortably without worrying about any slip-ups.

✳ Pay attention to those panties. If you like a certain cut in your undergarments, you'll most likely also like it as a bathing suit style.

Play with proportions. Standard black bikini not really doing it for you this year? Ditch your classic silhouettes and try a new cut. A high-

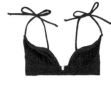

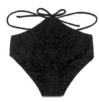

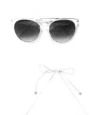

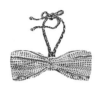

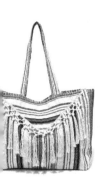

Don't waste precious vacation days on self-doubt. Relax. No one's perfect. Once you pick your suit, resolve to feel confident in your own skin.

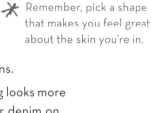

waisted two-piece or one with unique tie placements are personal favorites.

Mix and still match. Mix and match your bikini tops and bottoms for endless combinations.

Add a cover-up that you feel stylish in. Nothing looks more chic than a tunic; you can even wear this over denim on cool nights. A sarong can be worn a million ways (I love a dyed version), or go ahead and use that kimono we talked about in spring (see page 71).

Remember, pick a shape that makes you feel great about the skin you're in.

An oversized denim shirt makes for a cool beach cover-up option. I leave a few thin necklaces on at the beach and I throw it over my black suit when I get out of the water.

reflect

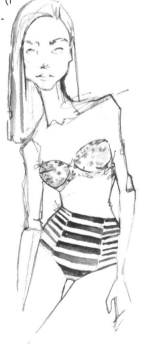

and then can i go to Santorini, though?

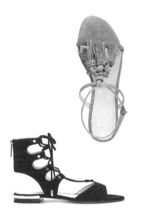

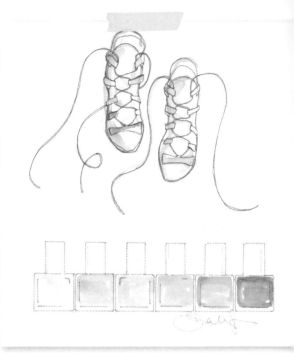

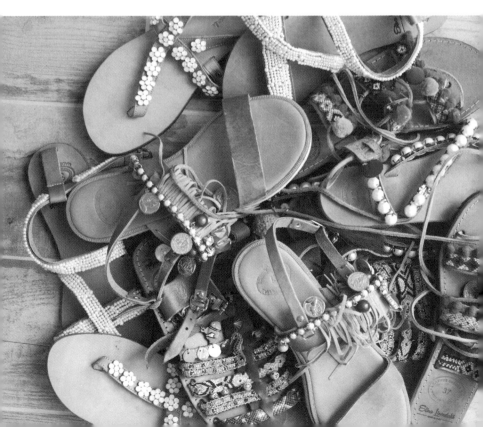

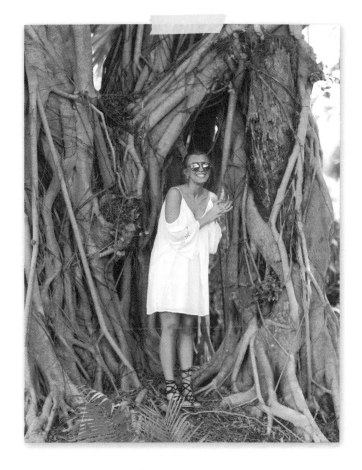

unleash your inner greek goddess

The ultimate sandal stock up—and the pedi shades to match.

I adore Greek sandals. (Hi. Elina Linardaki. For life.)

Because you are wearing just a few simple pieces for most of the summer heat, your sandals need to be taken seriously. Whether you are a simple strap-sandal girl or a laced-up Grecian goddess, here are a few flats to inspire you, and the pedi shades to perfect the look.

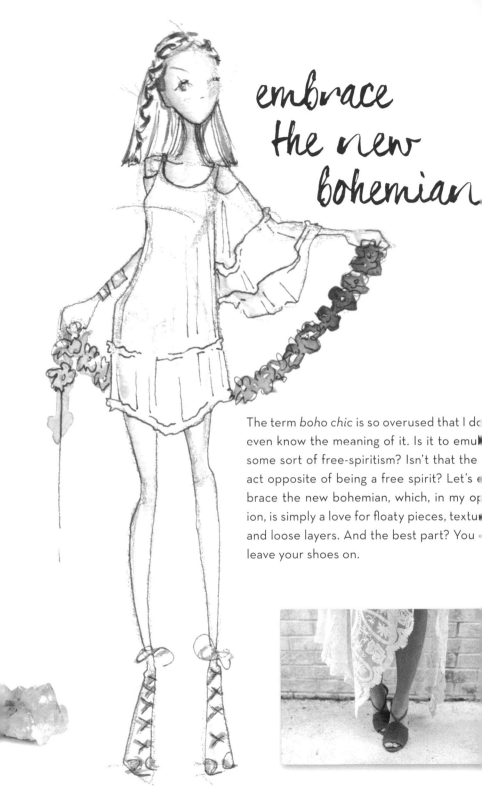

embrace the new bohemian

The term *boho chic* is so overused that I do[n't] even know the meaning of it. Is it to emu[late] some sort of free-spiritism? Isn't that the [exact] act opposite of being a free spirit? Let's [em]brace the new bohemian, which, in my op[in]ion, is simply a love for floaty pieces, textu[re] and loose layers. And the best part? You [can] leave your shoes on.

EASE IN

- A floaty cream top with embellishments (look for tassels, beading, coins) or really any top with a wide, flutter sleeve.
- Add a layer, a thin oversized sweater, or a sheer loose kimono top.
- Switch out your standard belt for a wide woven style. One with a tie front is even more fun.

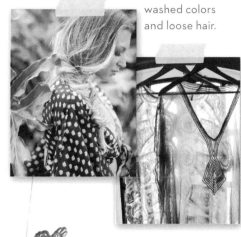

Keep your outfit cool with washed colors and loose hair.

STEP IT UP

- A fringed bag in a unique color hints at your carefree attitude.
- Trade in your tank for an ombré/dip-dyed version.
- Linen pants and V-neck tees worn together with a simple leather flat sandal feels breezy. Add a long necklace to make this feel more put-together.

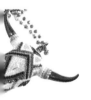

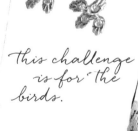

This challenge is for the birds.

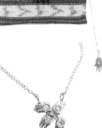

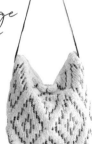

A loose fit is key here, so forget traditional sizing and wear what looks best.

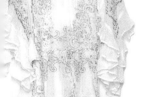

FEELING BRAVE

- Swap your standard sundress for a printed romper and sandals. I love mine covered with '90s florals.
- Rock a floppy straw hat with a floral top or a cozy wrap.
- A printed dress with long sleeves brings an element of romance to this look.

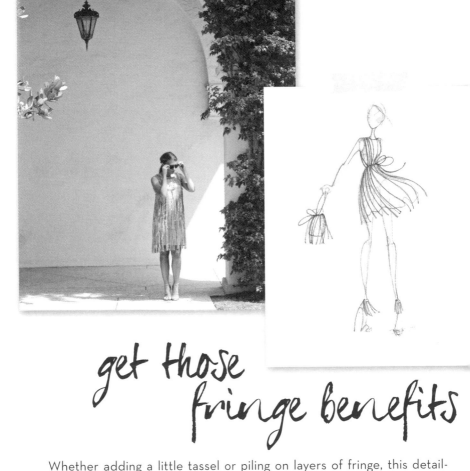

get those fringe benefits

Whether adding a little tassel or piling on layers of fringe, this detailing is such a playful element to add to an outfit mostly because of the way it moves with you. Put it on and you'll have the instant urge to jump around. Look ahead to our '70s challenge from Fall (page 142): you may have something in your closet worth bringing back out this summer. Fringe is forever.

EASE IN

- A keyfob tassel on a bag. No need to match it to your bag—choose any color you'd like.
- Shoes with small leather tassel detailing. I sport a classic penny loafer with my denim.
- Some Minnetonka booties with fringe around the top.

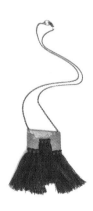

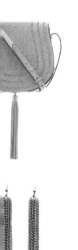

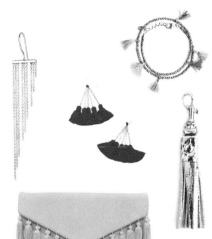

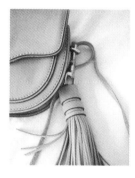

* Check out vintage shops for the most unique pieces.

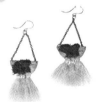

STEP IT UP

- Tassels on your jewelry. Such an easy way.
- Trim on a fitted skirt with strappy heels and a tank.
- A fringe purse or clutch—the longer the fringe the bolder the statement.

FEELING BRAVE

- A fringe jacket with a white tee and high-waisted jeans.
- A fringe maxi dress. Keep your hair sleek and let the piece stand for itself.
- Heels with fringe detailing around the ankle.

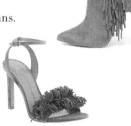

EASE IN

- Try pairing your chambray shirt (this is a staple) with black jeans.
- Play with different shades of denim. Dark jeans with a shirt in a lighter wash, or vice versa.

✳ Still too shy to get started? Look for a crisper denim top, and tuck it into some darker denim with a belt. Polished makeup completes the look.

STEP IT UP

- Wear differing washes in the same color (aka a top that feels like a worn or faded version of the jeans you have on).
- Dress this look up with a sleek nude heel.

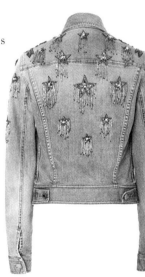

FEELING BRAVE

- Add a tailored jacket in a nice neutral over your shoulders to make this look feel sleek.
- Try some patchwork denim. It's exciting to push yourself out of your denim comfort zone.

{ reflect }

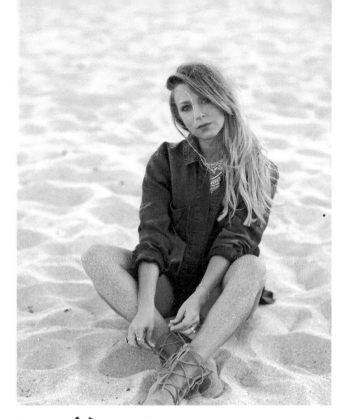

double down on denim

A denim button-down shirt over your favorite pair of jeans will have you looking cooler than a supermodel in an airport. There are three steps to pulling off the look:

1. Keep it very simple.
2. Less is more. *because this bears repeating.*
3. Just two denim pieces and very few accessories for the win.

Psst: No denim shoes, no denim hats needed—I'm talking about a top and a bottom here. Period.

perfect pairings
we go together like:

{ rock Tees x pearls }

A close-fitting vintage rock tee is best. Rhinestones are a cool sub if you aren't a pearl girl.

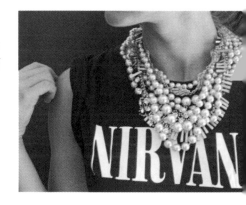

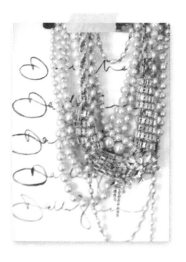

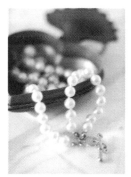

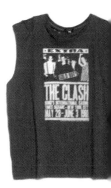

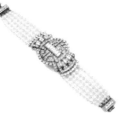

{ tee shirts x braids x studs }

I love a loose V-neck tee with a braided messy updo and a rhinestone stud earring. Pretty much my summer uniform.

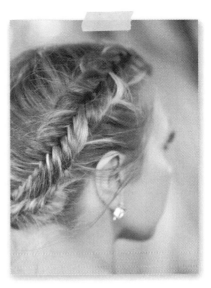

 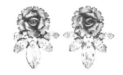

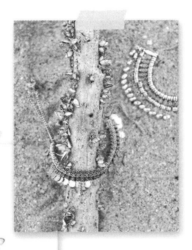

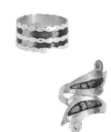

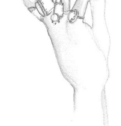

{ silver jewelry x sheer polish }

Stacks of silver rings look amazing next to sheer polish. Puts all the focus on your classic mani.

Design Your
Summer Palette

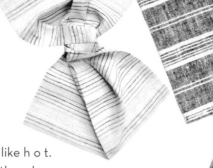

Spring ends fast, and now it's hot. No, like h o t.
In the summer sun I gravitate to weightless, breezy
silk tanks in lightweight colors with delicate straps. White, creams, and glistening golds begin to grace my hangers. I've packed away my regular blues and replaced them with extra-light washes with white splashes. After my rack is full of the simple lights, I bring in a few new colors in a mix of textiles. Relaxed tops that are faded and stitched fabrics in washed salmon fill the closet, followed by flowy bohemian embroidered tops in creams and dusty shades. All choices that will look even better next to those deep palm greens I've been filling my house with. Let's design your summer color palette.

My closet is beginning to look like an ice cream parlor. And I'm okay with that. Now it's time to create your own summer strategy. Place your notes or inspiration here:

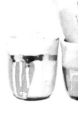

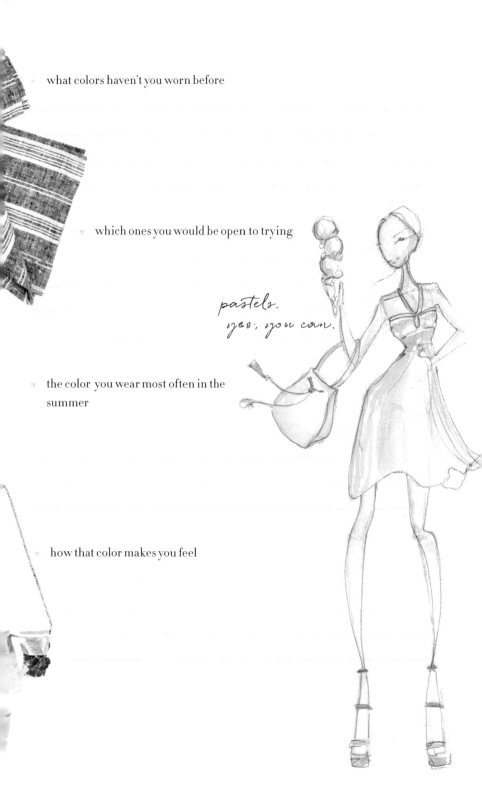

what colors haven't you worn before

which ones you would be open to trying

pastels.
yes; you can.

the color you wear most often in the summer

how that color makes you feel

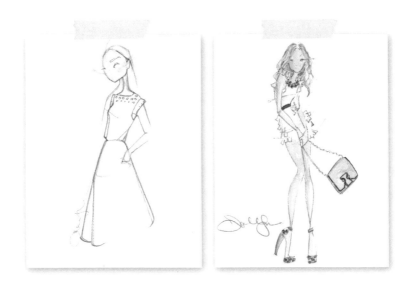

wear white without checking the calendar

One more fashion "rule" to throw out the window: that one that says there's a certain timeframe in which you should and shouldn't wear white. However, if any time is the time to rock an all-white look, it's right now in the sunshine. It won't draw extra heat to you, and nothing complements your tan better.

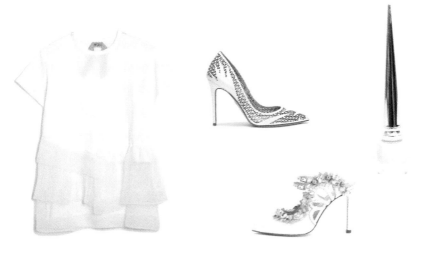

Just try it!

- Pair two textures to keep it interesting.
- Add layers for some depth.
- A two-piece white outfit looks chic.
- Keep it casual (white denim, white tee) with silver accessories and simple sandals.

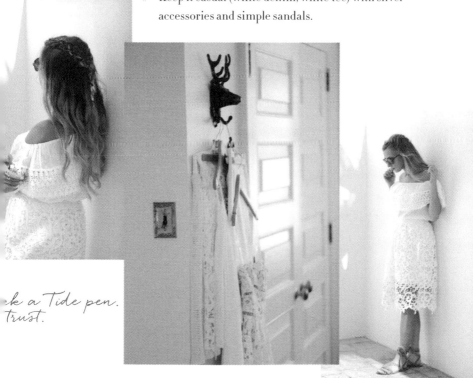

...k a Tide pen.
Trust.

Dusty rose, blush, berry, hues of peach—pink is a color that comes in such a sweet range of pigment. So why is the softest and sweetest color somehow the most intimidating to wear? I adore pink, and even I can see how some misdirected bubble-gum hues could turn you off the color. But with a bit of reeducation regarding the pink gradient, I assure you that you, too, can pull it off with ease.

i do believe you're blushing

✳ Sweep some sweet pink blush on the apples of your cheeks to completely change your complexion and take years off. But skip the pink lips with the blush, k?

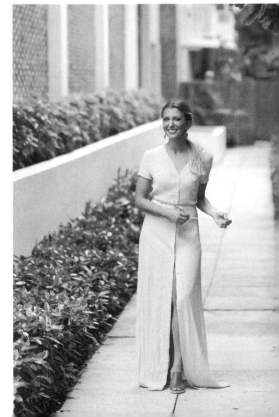

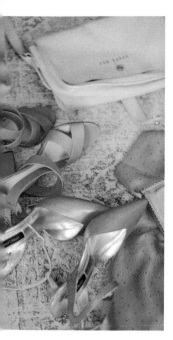

EASE IN

- A structured pink bag and a pink polish with some very fine shimmer. Complete the look with a pinky-brown lip and matching mani with a leather sandal.
- Add beige and/or a navy to a blushy pink top for a sophisticated look.
- Try a peach shade and pair it with a camel or brown suede.

 I like my pinks paired with browns and reds.

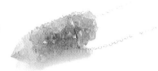

STEP IT UP

- Bright berry-pink dresses in silky fabrics. Look for floor length and long sleeves for a timeless option, and don't be afraid to match it with a deep berry lip.
- Pack some pink in your jewelry. I like a pink stone with a rough texture.
- Solid dusty-rose linen dresses pop up during the summertime. Pair with wedges, beach waves, sandy toes, and a tan. Look for an off-the-shoulder option or a unique cut for an extra-summery feel.

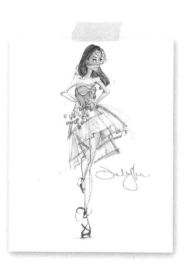

FEELING BRAVE

- Pair a bright berry-infused pink with a dash of red. I love a red pant with a berry top, or a red dress and a berry shoe.
- Channel your inner Floridian and add an unexpected green to your look.
- A dusty-rose baby doll dress; wearing this with a sleek middle part brought into a bun and sleek sunnies will keep it from looking too childlike.

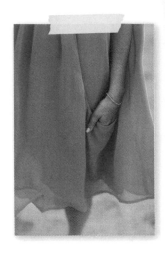

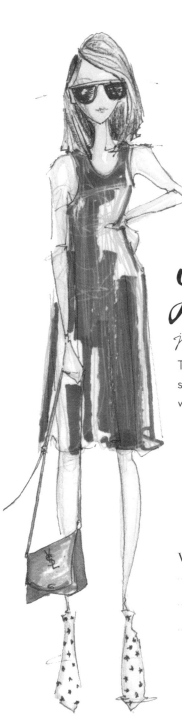

you glow, girl

just a leeeetle bit of neon.

This challenge is easier than you think: wear just the smallest touch of neon. Don't worry, a small amount won't have you looking like a walking highlighter.

What radiates from the depths of your closet?

....

....

....

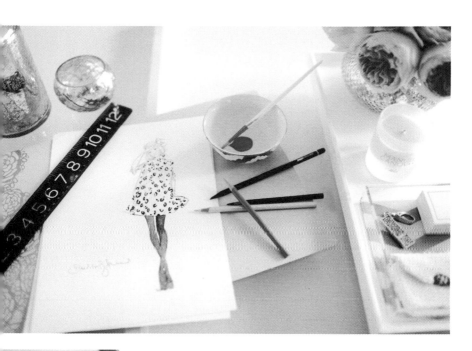

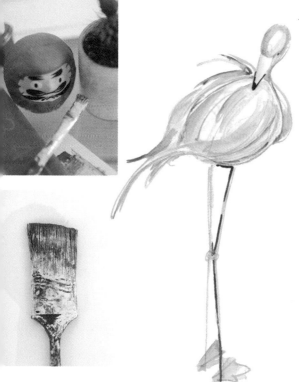

✳ Start with just the nails, a wallet that flashes only here and there. Then work your way up to a skirt, a shoe, or even a dress.

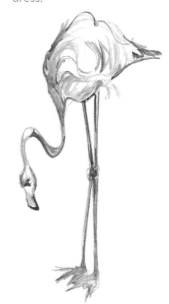

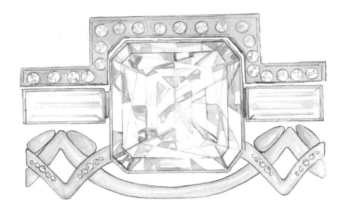

shine bright

If you were going to buy yourself a diamond ring, in a shape and a style that truly reflects you, what would it look like?

Ring shop online and think about what rings reflect your personal style. Because a diamond ring is such an investment, you are forced to overanalyze jewels and make definitive statements about the piece—and in turn about yourself—like: "I don't love that shape because it feels too modern for my taste." "I like an understated, simple ring." "Yes, this style is so 'me'!"

Regardless of whether it's a diamond, rhinestone, or vintage ring, the point is to wear a little bit more sparkle than you would today. This challenge is about adding a little sparkle and a lot of glamour to an average day.

What are some other ways you can do that using other aspects of your wardrobe?

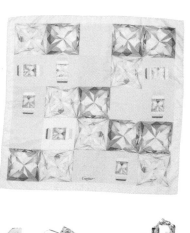

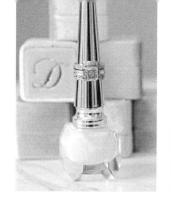

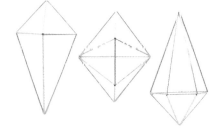

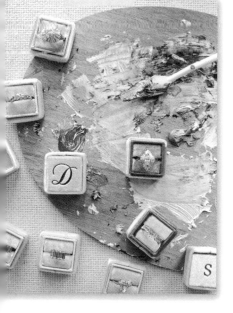

{ reflect }

....

....

....

get packing

They should have filmed all of *What Not to Wear* in the airport. It's filled with an awful mix of bad clothing that I'm forced to stare at for two whole hours before I board. Within that time, I've noticed that airport-goers seem to fall into one of three categories:

Category 1: People in their actual pajamas (ew).

Category 2: Women who are overly made-up, in some sort of bedazzled Ugg-leggings-hoodie combo. (Why?)

Category 3: The guy who's already dressed for his cruise even though it's snowing. Vacation starts when you arrive at your destination. (Take off your Tommy Bahama shirt and settle down.)

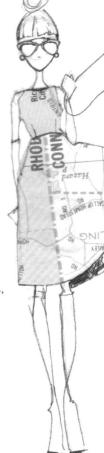

What these folks don't know—but you do *now*— is that the key to dressing for travel is wearing what you normally wear, in comfier, more casual fabrics. It's that simple.

Denim with a little stretch in it. An oversized scarf. A poncho. Flat booties. A jersey dress. Sneakers, slide-on shoes.

So, where are you off to? Doesn't matter.

What are you packing?

An oversized travel bag can go straight from the plane to the beach. I get my colorful embroidered bags from Nena & Co. and Lumily.

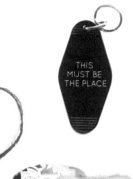

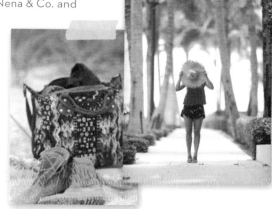

I travel alllllot for work, so I keep a half-packed bag ready at all times. Pack a small travel-ready bag with all your on-the-go essentials so you are prepped and ready to go on your next adventure at a moment's notice.

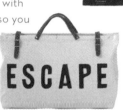

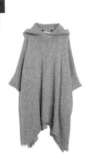

Here's my ultimate checklist that will have you covered for any sunny destination:

- ✓ lived-in jeans
- ✓ ankle-tie sandals
- ✓ travel bag
- ✓ small bag
- ✓ a few tees
- ✓ one pullover

- ✓ an airy dress
- ✓ one romantic top
- ✓ denim jacket
- ✓ swimwear
- ✓ sunnies

No vacation in sight? Pack a bag and make a day of it in the park. Staycations are just as fun if you have the right mind-set!

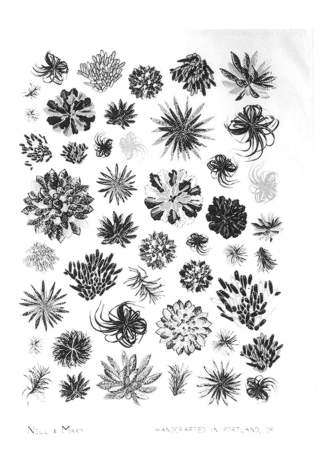

NELL & MARY   HANDCRAFTED IN PORTLAND, OR

southwestern summer vibes

The Southwest draws inspiration from Southern, Mexican, and West Coast cultures. Oh, and so do I. Add a little "Southwestern something" to your look today.

✳ This is done most easily with accessories.

EASE IN

- Metal feather accents in jewelry add a free-spirited feel to a light, lacy tank.
- Add a small cactus to your desk, windowsill, dining table . . . or if you're me, add seven.

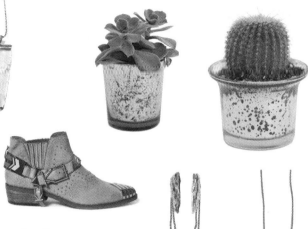

STEP IT UP

- A small silver buckle on a bootie or a belt.
- Piles of turquoise and flat silver jewelry. I collect these pieces on vacation and bring them back out every summer.

FEELING BRAVE

- Aztec print. I like this print on a large beach blanket or even on a bathing suit; it can also be a unique accent on an accessory.
- Embroidery in bright colors. Try this on a bag, a dress, or an off-the-shoulder top. It's always a stunner.

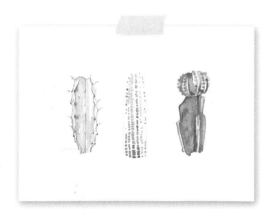

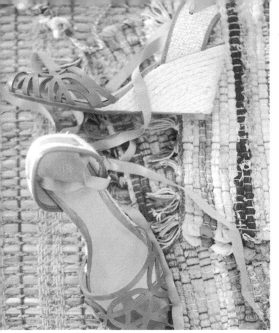

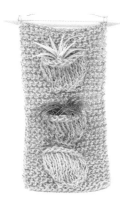

✳ Loving this challenge? A straw Panama hat is the easiest item to add to any of your summer looks.

something *wear woven*

What is it about summer that makes me want to break out the straw tote? I love me some wicker. There's something so carefree about a straw tote. It reminds me of flower market strolls and island vacations. Today, you're wearing something woven. The following suggestions work for all levels.

STRAW TOTE

Use a straw beach tote as your purse today, in any color that makes you happy. I like to keep a few hanging around the house (literally). They make amazing shop-ping totes. Warning: Carrying one of these might just convince you to pick up some fresh flowers during your errands.

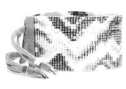

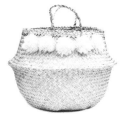

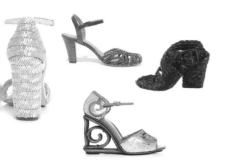

ESPADRILLES

Flat or wedge: makes no difference to me. If it is a shoe with a straw bottom, I'll buy it. All I know is I wore mine so much last summer that I nearly wore through the bottom. (True story.)

BRAIDS

Throwing a few quick braids in your hair is a simple trick to looking and staying cool in the heat. Plus, they look even better as they loosen up. Let the summer breeze perfectly muss your hair, then tuck any loose ends behind your ear and watch as your style gets better as the day goes on.

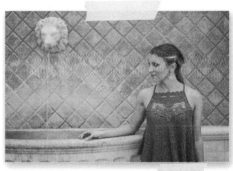

FRIENDSHIP BRACELETS

Why do we have to quit this accessory as adults? Thin, handmade braided versions work at any age because you are adding a small colorful pop to your summer staples in a casual way. Grab one while on vacation to remind you to loosen up a little. Have your niece or nephew make you one. Or two or three.

Or get a fancy version for yourself to jazz up your plain white tees.

 I wear a thin, hand-tied braided anklet all summer long.

throw some shade

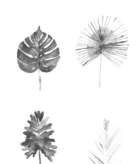

I've mentioned sunnies a number of times in challenge suggestions because they're an easy way to take your look up a level. Think you know what styles fit your face? Let's switch up your classic pair for a new shape. Here are the hottest ways to throw some shade this summer.

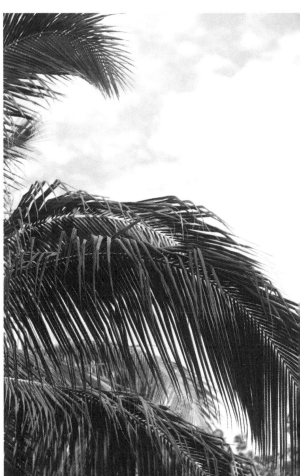

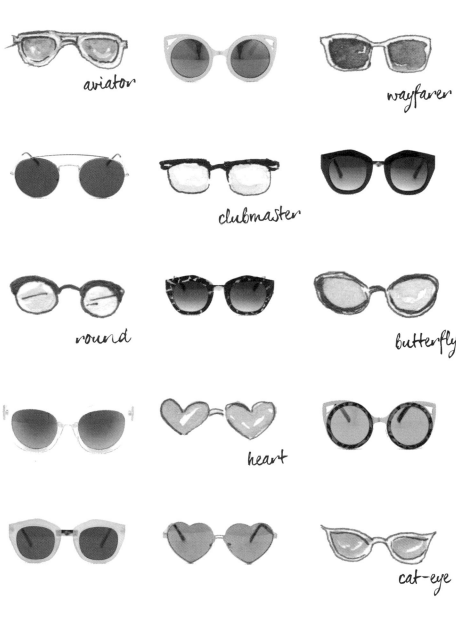

aviator

wayfarer

clubmaster

round

butterfly

heart

cat-eye

square

become a bronzed bombshell

So you love the sun—but you also love your skin. *good girl*. Thankfully, there are ways to stay warm and golden even though I'm addicted to my SPF.

Perfecting the golden glow isn't just about being tan; it's about warming up and accenting your skin to get a flattering, golden glow.

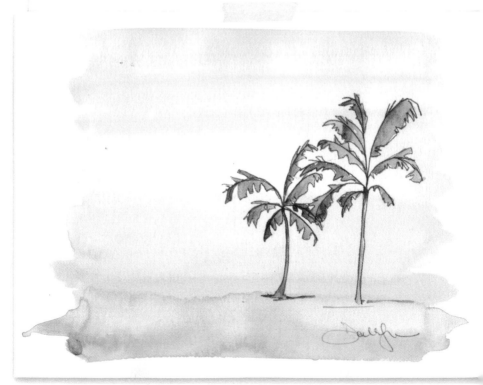

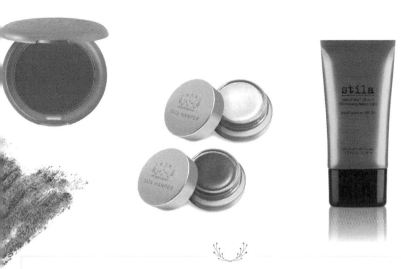

#THINGSWENEED

A contouring and highlight kit that includes cream bronzer and highlighter (I like Tata Harper's kit)
Powder bronzer (Estée Lauder's Bronze Goddess wins)

Translucent finishing powder (something like bareMinerals Mineral Veil)

1. Use your finger to apply the deeper shade (which should be two shades deeper than your skin color) to the hollow part of your face under cheekbones, the sides of your nose, and under your jawline.
2. Place the lighter cream down the center of your nose, on your chin, and under your eyes—on cheeks—to highlight. ✳ Don't forget your neck.
3. Blend.
4. Follow this up with a sweep of traditional powder bronzer. Give your face a nice once-over with a large brush.

After you are warmed up, set the look with a finishing powder. For a special night out you can even add an additional glow to your tan with the highlighter how-to on page 84.

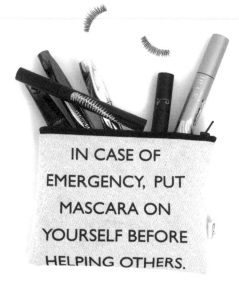

lash lust

Your eyes are the first thing people notice, and since makeup is so minimal in the summer, it's time to keep your fringe extra fab.

Mascaras make so many promises. It's important to know that not every mascara is alike and each formula/wand combo will produce a very different look.

Read the label, ladies. Mascara labels will tell you exactly what each does best: "Define." "Lengthen." "Thicken." All you have to do to get this right is 1) look at your own lashes and 2) read before you buy.

Wet formula = good for girls with already thick lashes,
because it defines.

Dry formula = nice for thinner lashes because it adds thickness.

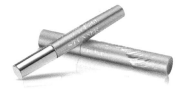

I personally like a drier mascara and my personal fave is Stila's HUGE extreme lash mascara. (It's all in the label.)

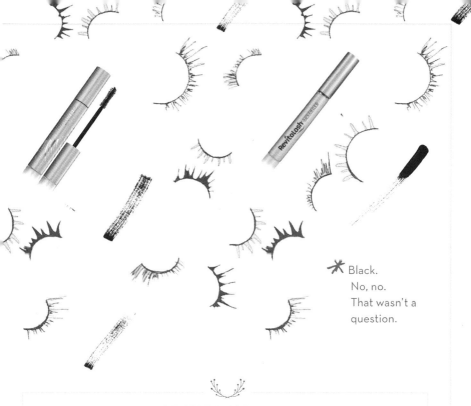

✳ Black.
No, no.
That wasn't a
question.

#OTHERTHINGSWENEED

Primer—helps the product go on
smooth

**Lash growth serums and
conditioner**—help with growth

Extensions—fun for a doe-eyed look
that lasts weeks

Eyelash comb—so you don't have
spidery clumps

False lashes—add a few singles to
the corners for an extra pop,
or go full length for a special
occasion

Eyelash curler—for extra oomph

Eye-makeup remover—because
it's important to care for the
lashes you have

Don't be afraid to combine two coats of different products to create
your own custom formula. I like my lashes long and thick, so sometimes I
layer two mascaras to get the job done. For duos I use CoverGirl's Lash-
Blast Length and then I add their LashBlast Volume. Brings the drama
every time.

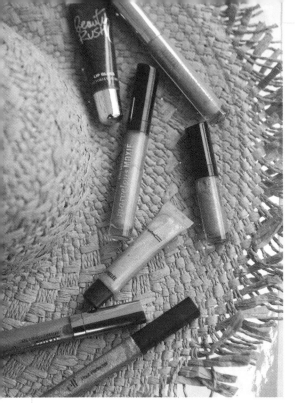

 bareMinerals glosses have jus[t] the right touch of shimmer—Flecks thin enough to catch light and subtle enough to keep you looking from like a preteen.

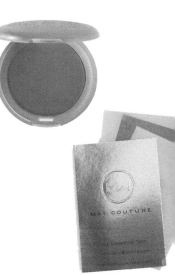

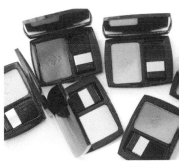 Lancôme for beautiful blush in all sorts of cheery shades.

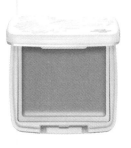

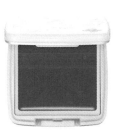

{ reflect }

give 'em the one-two punch

I have two beauty musts for summer: a bright blush and a shiny gloss. I keep a duo in my bag at all times so I can make sure I'm keeping my fresh-faced look late into the evening. As the long days take you on unplanned adventures, these two items are all you need in your bag for throughout-the-day touch-ups.

BOLD BLUSHES

The brighter, the better. Remember, they go on sheer. You'll be surprised at how flattering just a touch of bright pink, orange, or, dare I say, red blush can look. Use a big blush brush and keep these brights to a dusting.

SHIMMERY GLOSSES

A shimmery gloss goes a long way. The sun catches the sparks and keeps your smile shining even brighter than usual. I favor shades just darker than my natural lip color, and with a golden shimmer.

What shade would you like to try?

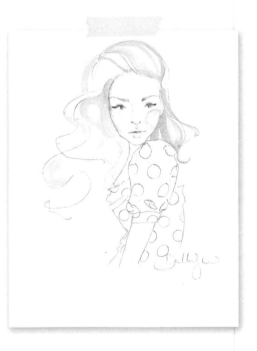

cheat on your moisturizer

"Put oil on my face? Oh, honey, no" was my exact reaction when a few years ago a makeup artist told me about facial oils. I have very sensitive skin, so no, and definitely no. It wasn't until I started working closely with Fresh cosmetics that I understood skincare a bit more and decided to try this out. I started a slow love affair with their Seaberry oil and slowly ventured out from there.

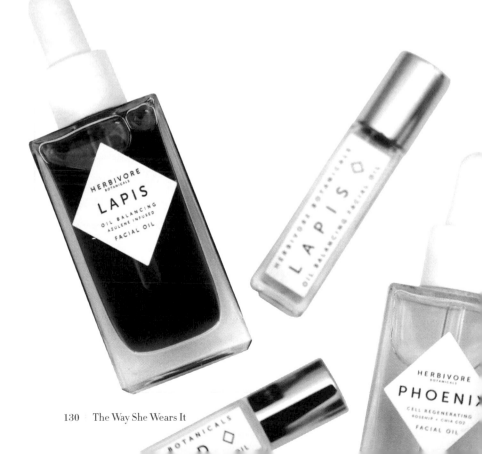

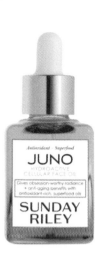
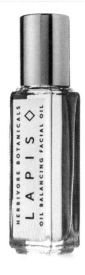
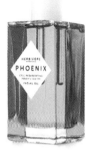
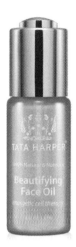

Two ways to get started:

1. Throughout the day, put a few drops on your palms, rub together, and press onto your face. For a second you look a little, well, oily—it's oil, people—but give it about 60 seconds and you have an instant cheeky glow. It's an easy way to freshen up and the amazing scent always gives me a recharge midday.

   Am I at a spa or am I at work right now?

2. Put a few drops in your moisturizer and apply to your neck and chest after a shower. Truth is, I actually started here and worked my way up.

   Softens.
   Smooths.
   Smells dreamy.

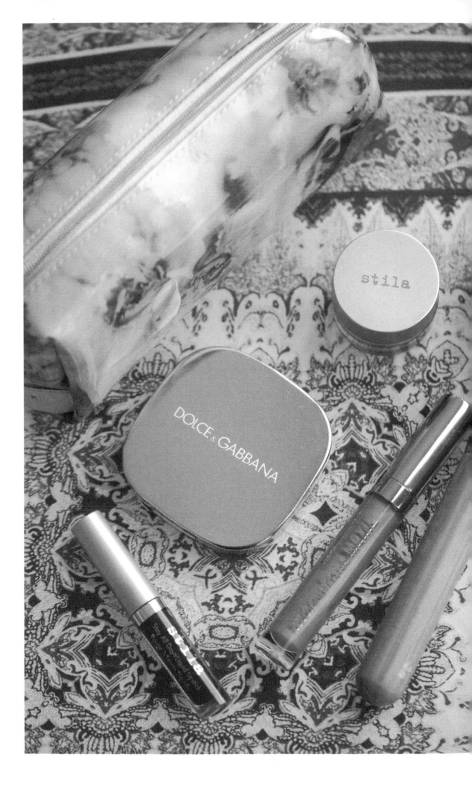

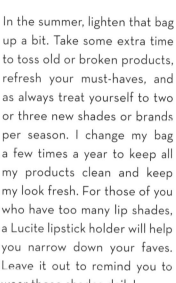

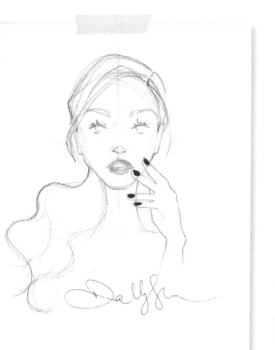

In the summer, lighten that bag up a bit. Take some extra time to toss old or broken products, refresh your must-haves, and as always treat yourself to two or three new shades or brands per season. I change my bag a few times a year to keep all my products clean and keep my look fresh. For those of you who have too many lip shades, a Lucite lipstick holder will help you narrow down your faves. Leave it out to remind you to wear those shades daily!

freshen up your summer makeup bag

#THINGSWENEED

Golden highlights	Apricot cream blush
Sunscreen	Bronzers
Long lashes	Natural nails
Beach-waved hair	

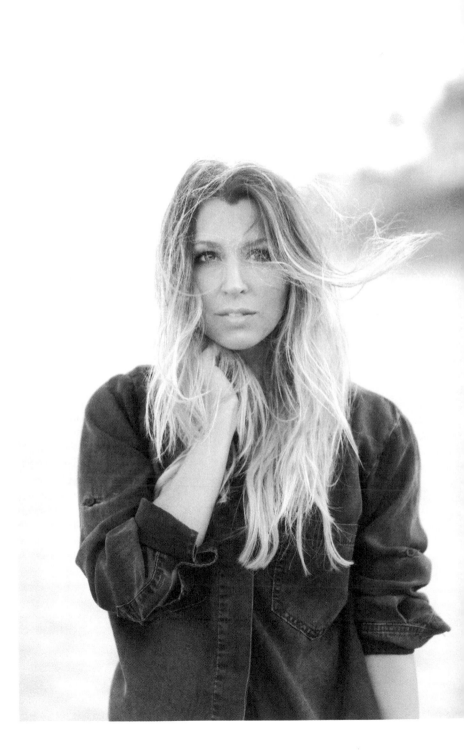

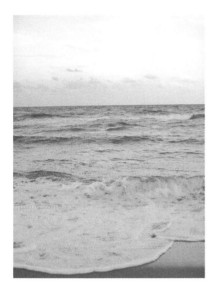
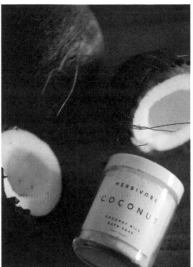

the challenge continues . . .

EMBRACE THE SIMPLE JERSEY SUNDRESS

You can get away with easy dressing in the summer, but you have to act on it. It's one single piece of clothing and makes you look put together, because it's a dress. How simple! Bonus: It feels comfier than a full look. Get after it

WRAP IT UP

A thin turban-inspired headband/wrap is very French looking in the summer. Throw it on at the beach to keep your hair back or channel your inner Audrey Hepburn and wear with a three-quarter-length sleeve.

BRING THE BEACH INSIDE

Choose some beachy scents and enjoy them when you are away from the waves. Coconut everything, sea salt hair sprays, and fresh-scented candles will let you enjoy the beach vibes when you can't be in the sand.

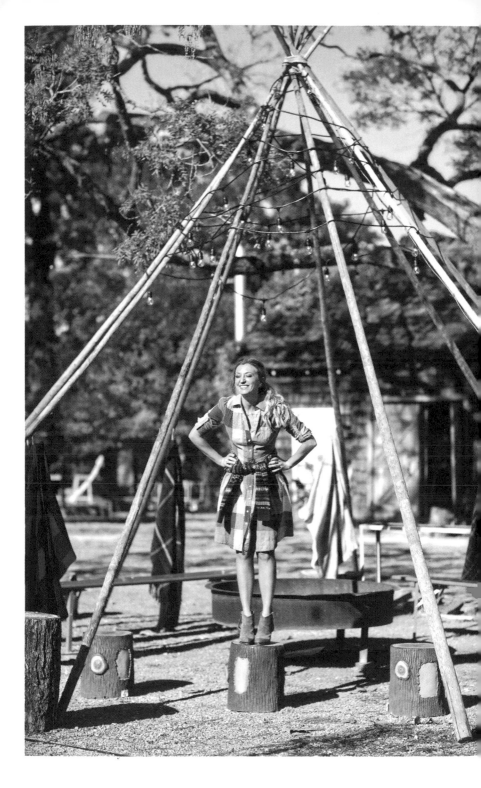

FALL

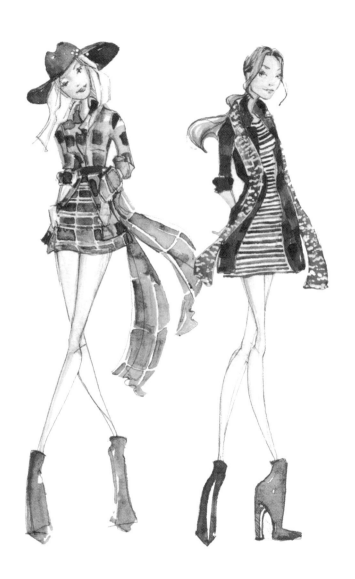

Attention, It girls: Along with a crisp breeze in the air, beanie weather has officially arrived. *How I've missed you, my jeans!*

It's time for the annual "unpacking of the sweaters" ceremony, during which I precisely unfold and tidy away the knits I had stored away for the summer, at which time, my life is made complete by coming across a jacket I forgot I even owned.

For the next few months, the usual dressing-for-temperature rules do not apply. I can wear sweaters and pants with open-toed heels. I get to wear multiple layers and still show a little bare leg. All this, and I'm still tan. *Sweet victory!*

Now that summer has ended, I'm craving polish and structure in my life. I begin by collecting a slightly embarrassing heap of September issues over which I pore in the same way I research visuals for a creative project—folding corners, ripping out pages, hanging page tears, circling accessories, and making lists. The result is a collage of images (worthy of being featured on a crime procedural) just waiting to be pieced together to reveal the answer.

There is a back-to-school feeling in the air. I have an urge to raid a college professor's closet for elbow-patched coats and vests. My office is already full of no. 2 pencils, but I have my eye on sleek leather backpacks and loafers.

Autumn comes and goes quickly, so grab your own collection of September issues and a caramel coffee and enjoy this style season while it lasts.

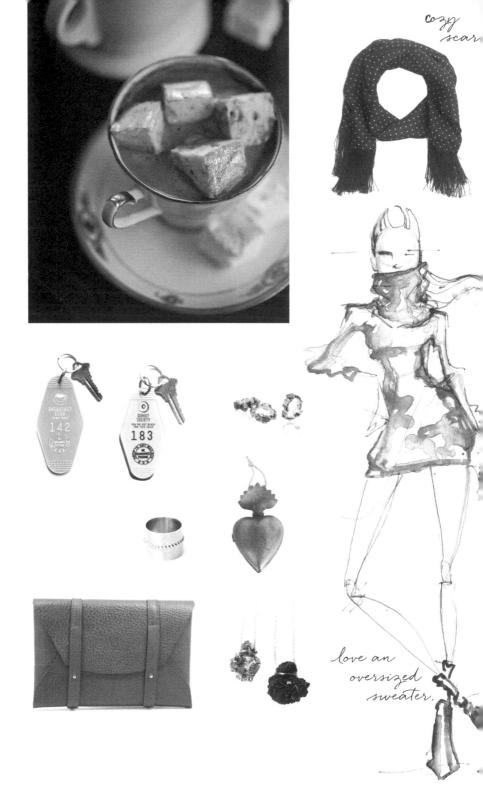

cozy
scarf

BREAKFAST
CLUB
142

DONUT
SOCIETY
YOU'RE NOT READY
FOR THIS JELLY
183

love an
oversized
sweater.

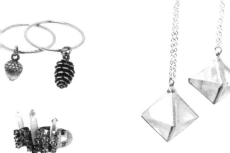

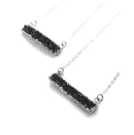

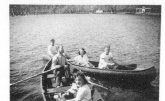
*field coats are kind
of my thing.*

#thingsweneed

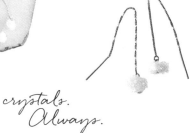

*candles x indie music
x camp socks*

MOONLIGHT
MILE

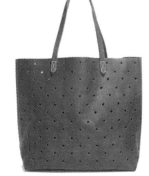

*crystals.
Always.*

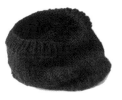

✳ Take this look to your hair with
   a middle part with the sides
   curled away from your face.
   Think more Sienna Miller and
   less Farrah Fawcett.

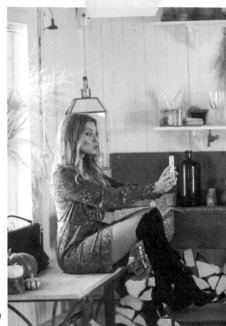

bring back
that '70s chic

Fashion in the '70s had a tailored vibe that is timeless. Something about fall makes it feel like the right time to get a little extra fitted. For me, once the weather drops, I practically live in a pair of curator pants (semipleated in the front and thinned out at the ankle). Today, you'll add something '70s inspired to your outfit, even if it's only a single touch. Don't worry, you won't look like you're headed to a costume party. By keeping the rest of your look modern, you'll avoid looking too far-out. *Dig it.*

EASE IN

- A large round pair of sunglasses.
- Wide-leg pant with a belt.
  Both thick or thin belts work here.
- A button-front skirt in denim or suede.
- Corduroys. (These don't have to bell. Grab them in your normal cut.)

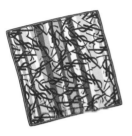

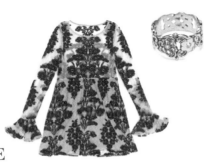

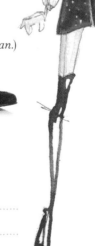

FEELING BRAVE

- A men's-style vest. *Annie Hall dared me to.*
- A printed silky dress worn over a collared shirt or with a schoolboy blazer.
- A long, floral dress paired with boots that you only see when you strut your stuff.
- Add a fringed jacket.

STEP IT UP

- Over-the-knee boots. (No—I repeat, no—tight miniskirts allowed with this. You've seen *Pretty Woman*.)
- Suede shoes.
- Something cream and crocheted.
- A printed silk shirt.

reflect }

....

....

....

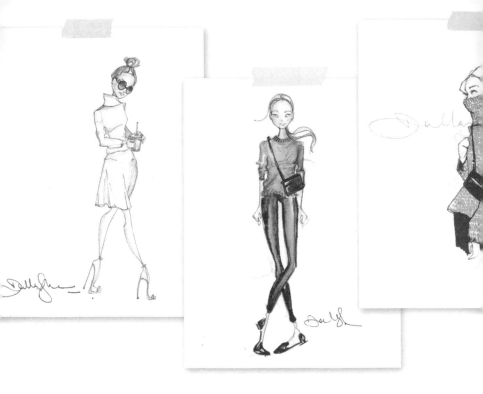

embrace
the Sweater weather

If you're like me, you own a million sweaters (thanks, J.Crew for making me believe I need every single cashmere sweater you produce, year after year). But when it's cold in the morning and you get out of your warm bed, you throw on the first sweater you reach for and pair it with the jeans you wore yesterday. You then add the all-too-common flat boot and you are out the door. Nothing wrong with that—oh, except for *snooze-fest*! Today's challenge is to embrace your sweaters. I love my sweaters cozy and oversized and paired with fancy flats.

Here are ten other ways to turn this
staple into something more:

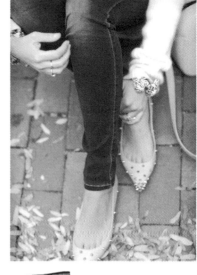

1. Your fitted printed favorite? Tuck it
    into a long skirt or over a dress.
2. Your solid classic? With a matching
    overcoat, ankle jeans, and heels.
3. Your really-oversized-but-extra-cozy?
    With leather leggings.
4. Your thin crewneck? With a fitted
    black midi skirt and booties (sans
    tights).
5. Your long boxy turtleneck?
    With a lace slip skirt.
6. Big and blouse-y? With a
    cross-body bag to define
    your figure.
7. Your men's-style sweater?
    With a flowing midi skirt
    and heels.
8. Your old cable knit? With
    shorts, sneakers, and a
    men's watch.

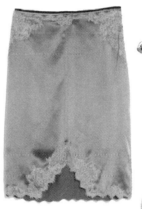

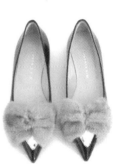

9. Your cashmere turtleneck?
    With a necklace over top and your hair tucked in. Add
    that overcoat here for an extra dose of chic.
10. Your holiday staple? With
    distressed denim and
    strappy, festive heels.

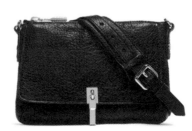

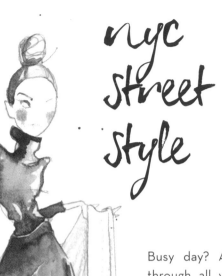

nyc street style

Busy day? All black can get you through all your errands flawlessly. Take a message from the Big Apple today. Throw on head-to-toe black, grab your keys, and hit the streets.

_____ is the new black.

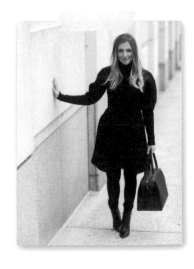

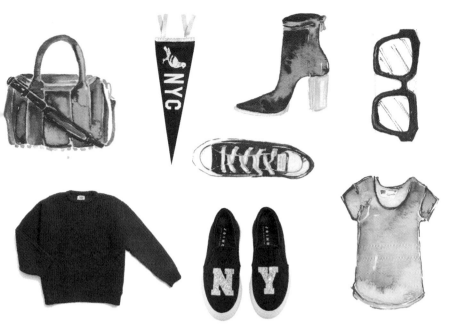

Why you *think* New Yorkers wear black: "Because it's professional?"

Why New Yorkers *really* wear black:

1. They are busy and it's easy.
2. It looks put together when you can't decide what to wear in the morning.
3. It's foolproof and appropriate for anywhere those hectic city days take you. From creative meetings to after-work rosé with the ladies to fashion-week front rows.
4. It's always the appropriate time of day to wear black.
5. It's never trendy.
6. You're semi-intimidating, in a cool way. *Don't even think about saying my outfit needs a "pop of color."*
7. Black is universally flattering: No matter what your skin tone or body type, you're good.

re you from NYC?
o, but my wardrobe is.

new york

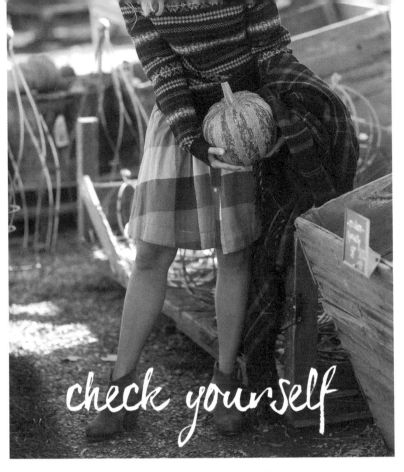

check yourself

The power of plaid. One pattern to unite golfers, hipsters, preppies, and '90s celebs. Plaid is proof that the way you wear it speaks volumes about you. *Hey, someone should write a book about that* . . . There's something for everyone in this challenge, whether you've been avoiding it or have so much of it you don't know what to do with it.

EASE IN

- An oversized plaid scarf with jeans and a solid tee.
- Plaid shoes with black slim-cut ankle pants or jeans and basically anything else.
- A thick-knit plaid mini with tights, an oversized sweater, and a leather backpack.

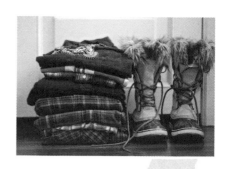

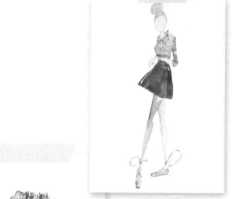

TEP IT UP

A fitted and ladylike plaid dress with bare legs and heels.

Plaid wide-leg pants worn with a tie-bow blouse, a chunky heel, a middle part, and an attitude.

A plaid blazer will keep you professional and still on trend. Pair it with riding gloves for your commute and a color-block clutch.

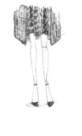

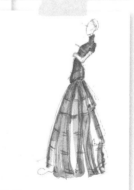

FEELING BRAVE

Search for a long plaid maxi for MAXImum impact. *See what I did there?*

A plaid midi skirt with a crisp white top tucked in and leopard heels.

A large wooly plaid coat draped over your shoulders with a dress underneath. Bonus: Throw on some patent Mary Janes for a street-style moment.

blazers outside the office

Blazers are not just a work staple. Sure, they're associated with professionals, but with the variety of colors, sizes, and fabrics available, there is a blazer out there for everyone. For today's challenge, get your blazer out of the cubicle and into the street.

 My go-tos are a long but slim camel wool, a light gray schoolboy with gold buttons, and a boxy black double-breasted.

* Try a plaid or herringbone. I wear my printed versions as a coat in the fall.

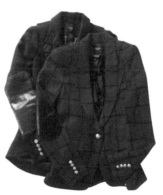

{ *reflect* }

....

....

....

EASE IN

- Worn as a coat, with an oversized scarf, distressed denim, and shades. (If the jacket and scarf are both prints, this can take the look up a notch.)
- Over a fitted sweater with a structured but deep bag.
- With cuffed jeans, a T-shirt (no tight tanks here, please), and a men's watch.

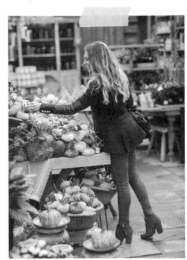

STEP IT UP

- A navy or gray worn over a hooded sweatshirt, with a statement necklace. (I wear my blazers one size up for this reason.)
- The same slightly oversized navy, worn belted and with dark denim. Push up those sleeves for the perfect touch.

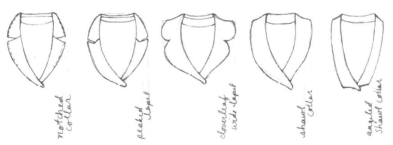

notched collar   peaked lapel   cloverleaf wide lapel   shawl collar   angled shawl collar

* You're looking for something special here, not a blazer that can be mistaken for a suit jacket. Seek out interesting textures and collars, as well as special details like patches and beautiful buttons.

FEELING BRAVE

- Worn over a maxi dress with booties. This is a nice way to transition your summer clothing in the fall.
- Wrapped and belted over a shorter, fitted knee-length dress and heels.

the secret to looking parisian chic

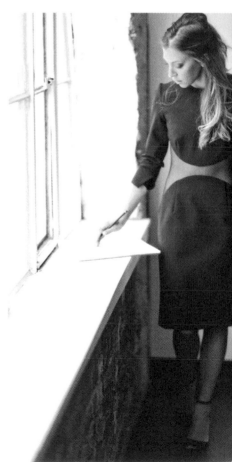

. . . is minimalism. Sometimes looking effortlessly chic means forgetting the details and keeping things sleek and minimal. All you'll need is a few articles of clothing with good lines, and in solid colors, and you'll radiate that je ne sais quoi. As the French say, "Less is more." This is a lesson in how good tailoring can actually make your clothes look much more expensive. When combined, neutrals in classic cuts look chic in a very casual I-just-threw-this-on type of way. It's the least complicated outfits that have the strongest impact.

> Peruse websites like Zady, Everlane, and Zara for inspiration on how to get this look right.

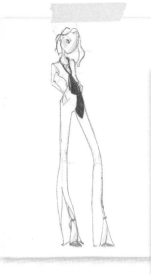

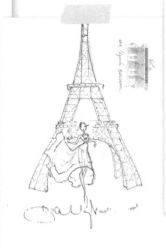

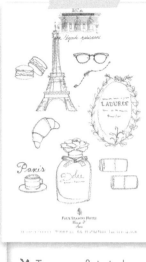

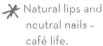

✳ Natural lips and
   neutral nails –
   café life.

✳ Try some flats today.
   Easy for walking on
   those cobblestone
   streets.

Head to your closet and follow these steps:

1. Start by looking for solid-colored clothing with clean lines in
   gray, black, white, cream, taupe, and denim.
2. Choose two or three colors and narrow down your options.
3. Keep your outfit simple: a top, a bottom, sleek shoes, and a
   solid bag with simple lines.
4. Skip the jewelry, but if you simply cannot,
   then very thin, delicate pieces only
5. Go light on the makeup. Matte, natural, and
   fresh, with a nude lip (page 53). Add a sweep
   of bronzer to your cheekbones to warm up a
   bit if you need to. I also love a strong brow here.

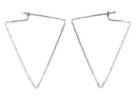

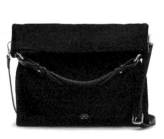

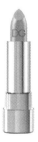

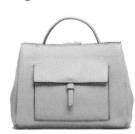

si jolie

live on the edge

Chances are you already have a leather (or faux-leather) jacket in your closet from before this book or from when you raced to the store after you read the NYC street style challenge on page 146. If you still don't have a black leather jacket, it may be time to rethink why that is . . . it wasn't until I started traveling so often that I realized how important a black leather jacket is. You can throw it on over anything, wear it anywhere, and it's great between seasons when you can't predict the temperature.

keep on

Zipper details.

how i wear mine

1. With my black jeans, a sweater, and studs.
2. With a loose, striped long-sleeve shirt.
3. Over a tucked-in standard gray turtleneck, with a long gold necklace and a belt.
4. Over a spring dress with a dark winter scarf.
5. With boots and a long, pleated maxi skirt.
6. Over my shoulders with a patterned sweater underneath and a clutch.

how you wear yours

1.
2.
3.
4.
5.

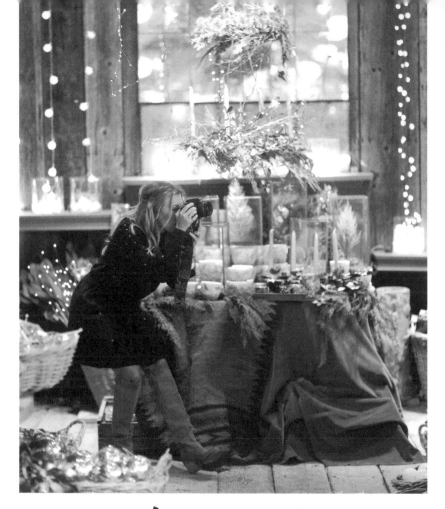

go sole searching

In the fall, your boots are probably the items in your closet you wear most, second only to your jeans. You add them to every look as an afterthought, so it makes sense to collect wear-with-everything styles. Boots are not inexpensive, which is why you need to make your selections carefully, but they last forever—so long as you take care of them—and most look better with wear. My favorite boots are taupe knee-highs that almost qualify as over-the-knee, aaaaand I've had them for seven years. Truth.

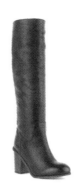

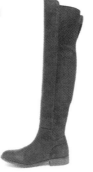

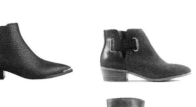

You can spray your boots with a weather-resistant spray to keep them shinier longer. I tend to keep my heeled boots polished and embrace the wear on my flat styles.

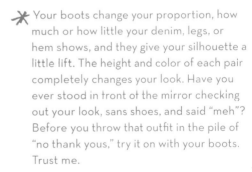

The Only Three Pairs of Boots You'll Ever Need

1. **Knee-high boots.** Flat and heeled. (I personally love brown and caramel shades.)
2. **Booties.** Flat and heeled. (I always keep flats in black and a brownish-gray.)
3. **Heeled over-the-knee boots.** Thin and chunky heels. (Black is my must-have for this style.)

Your boots change your proportion, how much or how little your denim, legs, or hem shows, and they give your silhouette a little lift. The height and color of each pair completely changes your look. Have you ever stood in front of the mirror checking out your look, sans shoes, and said "meh"? Before you throw that outfit in the pile of "no thank yous," try it on with your boots. Trust me.

Just because they're the only ones you'll ever need doesn't mean you're limited to three pairs total. Collect these carefully over the years in as many colors, heel types, and heights as you deem necessary.

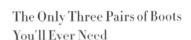

Therapy Check-in

So . . . how are you?

Take some time again to ask yourself how all these fall challenges are going.

Are you feeling more poised in all those plaids?

1. WHAT'S ONE WORD THAT DESCRIBES YOUR PERSONAL STYLE TODAY?

2. DOES WHAT YOU'RE WEARING TODAY MAKE YOU FEEL GOOD?

3. WHAT'S ONE THING YOU ARE BEGINNING TO UNDERSTAND ABOUT YOUR PERSONAL STYLE?

4. WHAT ARE YOU ENJOYING LEARNING ABOUT YOURSELF DURING THIS PROCESS?

5. WHAT DO YOU NEED TO TAKE MORE TIME FOR IN ORDER TO LIVE YOUR MOST STYLISH LIFE?

6. ARE YOU TAKING THE TIME YOU PROMISED YOURSELF?

7. ARE YOU TAKING TIME TO ENJOY THE BEAUTIFUL THINGS AROUND YOU?

Keep on.

Reward yourself by doing something nice for yourself. I think you deserve it. A trip to the pumpkin patch? A new pair of driving gloves? What will it be?

perfect pairings
we go together like:

{ *socks* x *mocs* }

Why so serious? If you're staying home
and playing board games
by the fire, why not throw
on not one, but two of
your most comfortable
things? *How-hygge!*

{ *bare legs*
         x *booties* }

Different dress/skirt lengths work
with different bootie/boot lengths.
Try various pairings and see which
you like best.

{ *Tweed*
  x *herringbone* }

Pair. Up. The. Prep.

Design Your Fall Palette

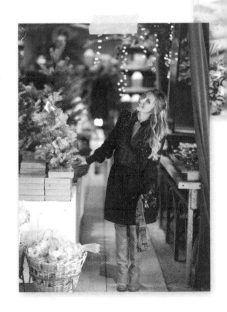

Fall fashion season is the time I take self-reinvention most seriously. And why not? Even the trees are outfitted in new colors. Shouldn't we be, too? My color palette differs slightly from the fiery golds and oranges on the trees outside. I wear a lot of warm cream, black, light grays, camel, dusty pinks, and dashes of rust. Then I bring in new colors with my flannels, plaid blazers, and silk prints. Caramel-colored hats, brown lip shades, and peachy silk shirts fill my drawers. I wear lots of muted textures: herringbone, tweed, and tortoiseshell.

Black Swiss dots and shiny chocolate oxfords complete my palette, and I'm ready to fill the house with millions of teeny white pumpkins.

It's time for your fall rebrand.

It's time to create your own fall rebrand. Place your notes or inspiration here:

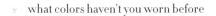 what colors haven't you worn before

which ones you would be open to trying

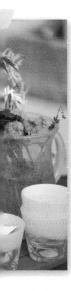

the color you wear most often in the fall

*if you said marigold
we're probably
best friends.*

how that color makes you feel

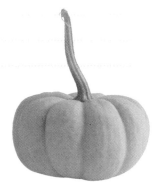

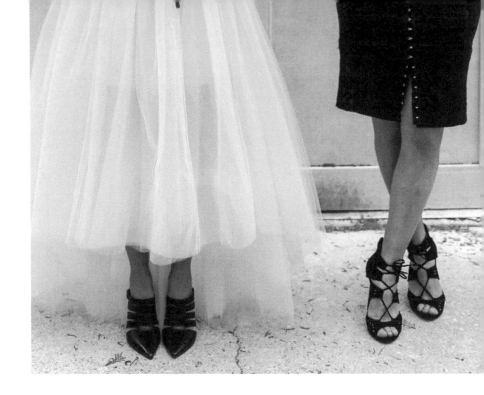

cream meets black

One of my favorite color combos in the fall is cream and black. It doesn't really matter how you pair the two; the warm white always complements the intensity of a cool black tone. And the best part? This challenge is easy to ace since you already own pieces in these colors.

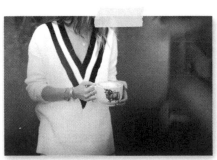

I'll take a large black with extra cream.

✻ Try this look with a winged black eyeliner.

EASE IN

- Black jeans, oversized cream sweater, ring stacks, and black booties.
- A top or dress with a cream-and-black print.
- Cream top, black quilted bag, and sunnies.
- Cream cable-knit turtleneck, dark skinny jeans, black heeled booties.

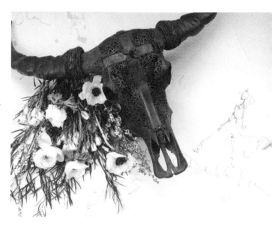

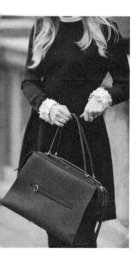

STEP IT UP

- Take it outside with a cream coat and a black scarf, or black coat and a cream scarf.
- Black moto pants, silk cream button-down, oversized clutch tucked under your arm.
- All black with a cream coat.
- Cream skirt that hits midcalf, worn with black booties.
- All black with a cream knit hat and a rosy cheek.

FEELING BRAVE

- Short lace cream dress with black booties.
- All cream clothing with a large-brimmed black hat.
- Cream dress, cream coat, cream shoes, cream-and-black bag (reddish-brown lip and lots of black mascara).
- Cream sleeveless turtleneck sweater, fishtail braid with a black ribbon on it.

* Want a little something more? Add a rich nail color or a brown bag.

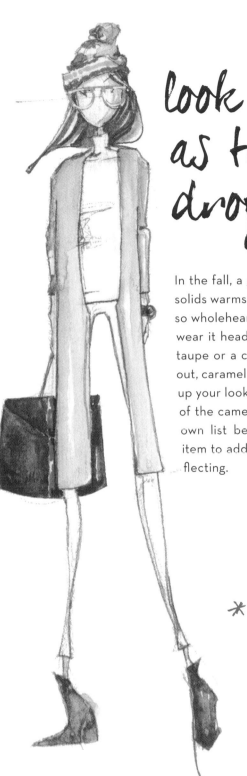

look warm as the temp drops

In the fall, a golden-camel shade added to solids warms up the skin a bit. I believe this so wholeheartedly that on occasion, I even wear it head to toe. While wearing a light taupe or a cool beige can often wash you out, caramel instantly warms and sweetens up your look. To guide you, I've made a list of the camel pieces I own. Continue your own list beneath, and then choose one item to add to your look today before reflecting.

✳ Pair different shades of camel together and add a blush tone to the mix.

1. A trench coat *perennially chic*
2. Classic tee—an essential layering piece
3. A floor-length belted wool coat
4. Leather skirt (this shade is unexpected and works well with prints)
5. I own one cardigan *It's a very lightweight cropped camel*
6. Cashmere sweater (Caramel-based animal print? Even better.)
7. Woven leather bag *looks even better with age*
8. Suede shirt-jacket
9. A longline mohair duster
10. Heels (a warm camel tone instantly warms all skin tones)
11. A felt hat
12. Faux-fur scarf
13. Cable-knit turtleneck poncho
14. A slightly deeper shade of camel pants
15. Suede button-front skirt
16. Grandpa sweater, cardigan-style, complete with rounded dark brown buttons *imma take your grandpa's style*

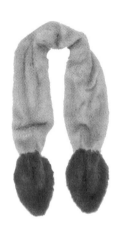

✳ Extend the tanned look to your makeup. A deep russet blush and a gloss will take this look from warm to hot.

✳ Swap out your standard black umbrella for a camel shade with a long, deep-brown hooked handle. You might even look forward to a rainy day.

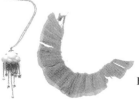

get wild

Animal print is the one challenge I can pretty much guarantee the response to: some kind of a face. Sometimes a client gives me a raised eyebrow, sometimes it's a head tilt of uncertainty, and sometimes it's full-on smush-face. So go ahead, get the eye-rolling out of your system before you start this challenge. When worn correctly, animal print holds the power to make you look expensive and intriguing. When chosen carelessly, the only thing it will make people wonder is where you're stopping on the way to a Vegas bachelorette party.

This trick to wearing animal print right lies in the *shape* and the *print*.

SHAPE

When shopping for animal print, seek out classic items with strong, sharp lines. Stick to classic silhouettes, avoid the tricky print in quirky shapes, and steer clear of flashy colors at all costs.

Should I wear an animal print shift dress? *yes.*

Isn't this pink zebra print so cute? *nope, it's not.*

Can I try on this cape coat? *yes.*

Purple was my sorority color, so I'm really feeling this purple print. *put it down right now.*

Will I get enough wear out of this structured clutch? *yes.*

Ruffled bag? *no.*

Platform heels? *skip.*

> ✳ Tight material is a no, tighter print is a yes. Prints where the spots are smaller and placed closer together are more flattering.

Spaghetti straps? *no, look for sleeves, please.*

Pointed-toe heels? *buy immediately.*

Ooh, feels comfy, is this jersey? *slowly back away from the stretchy material.*

PRINT

Animal print should vary in both the background color and the foreground pattern itself. Stay away from anything without depth (aka, that looks like it could be a wrapping paper). Which one of these is worthy of your closet?

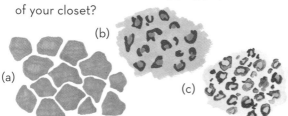

(a)

(b)

(c)

If you picked c, and only if you picked c—you are now free to shop.

EASE IN

✳ Wear animal print discerningly. There's no way to wear zebra print head to toe and not look like a zebra.

- A leopard clutch or pointed-toe heels are your new best friends.
- Pajamas or a silk robe.

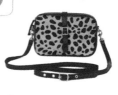

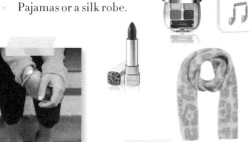

STEP IT UP

- Wear an animal-print shift dress with bare legs, heels, and a sleek pony.
- Pair a printed top with a strong eyeliner. *(bonus points if you wink at someone.)*

FEELING BRAVE

- Pair with another print. Try a spotted cape coat for a wow factor.
- Swap the standard leopard print for something more fun, like Dalmatian dots.

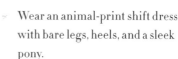

look
california cool

The cheapest accessory in your closet is also the one that can make you look instantly cooler: the beanie. Once a homeless staple turned key piece to a California cool look. Black, grays, and cream colors are easy to wear with anything equally easy to find. This inexpensive accessory is my off-day must have. It's noon and I've earned the right to stay on my couch for the entire day. My hair is 99% dry shampoo, I'm not in the mood for an official "look" today, but I do have a few things to do. Grab keys. Add beanie.

THREE STEPS TO THE MOST FLATTERING FACE FRAMING

1. Loosely and quickly part your hair in the middle.

2. Pull your hair forward in front of your shoulders.

3. Add beanie.

Pom removed = instant chill factor

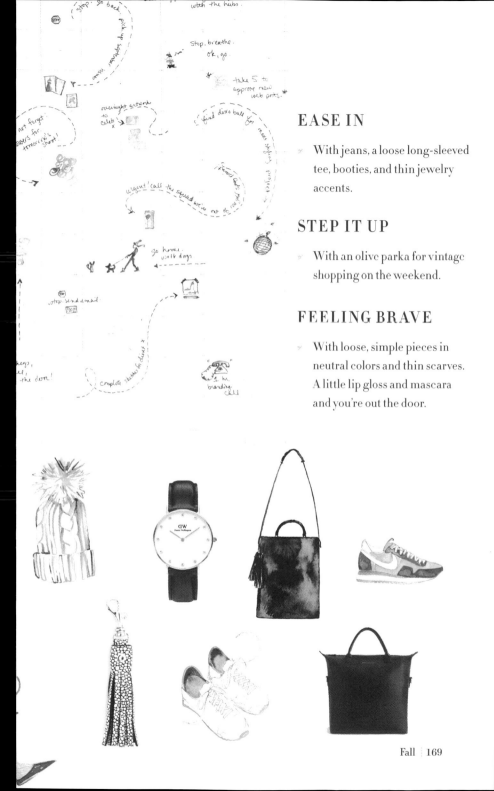

EASE IN

⚬ With jeans, a loose long-sleeved tee, booties, and thin jewelry accents.

STEP IT UP

⚬ With an olive parka for vintage shopping on the weekend.

FEELING BRAVE

⚬ With loose, simple pieces in neutral colors and thin scarves. A little lip gloss and mascara and you're out the door.

don't overthink
this look.

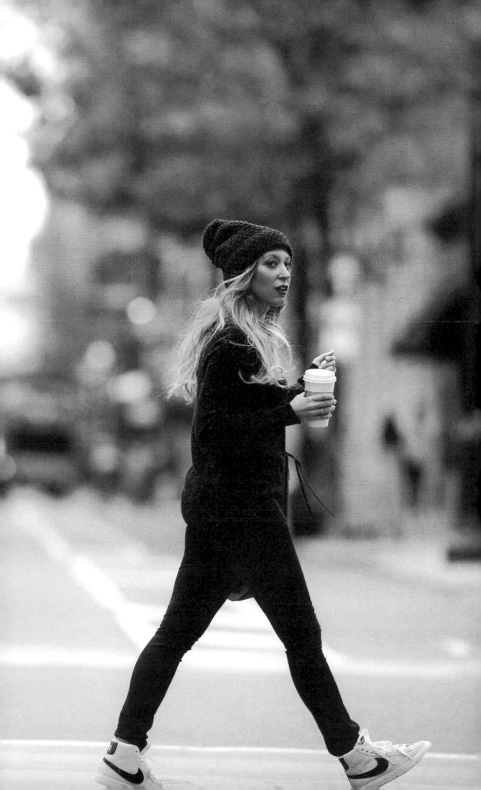

mix up masculine and feminine for a boyish charm

All you have to do for this challenge is mix and match. Think of it as a matching game. Add your fave masculine and feminine pieces to the following lists and then mix!

FEMININE	MASCULINE
Thin heels with a double strap	Glasses with thick frames
Piles of bracelets	Oxfords
Cat-eye sunglasses	Men's watch
Midi skirt	Boyfriend jeans
Floral pencil skirt	Men's-style striped button-downs
Pastel dresses	Men's belt
Pink nail polish	Boyfriend jacket
Braided hair	Field vest
Bright lips	Bow tie
Bowed flats	Tweed jacket with elbow batches
Something sequined	Tuxedo jacket
Anything with ruffles	Suspenders
Rhinestone accents	Camp socks
Delicate scarf	Loafers
Statement earrings	Converse

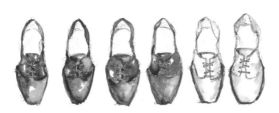 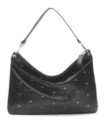

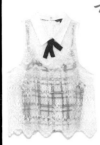

✳ Keep an eye open for masculine pieces in feminine colors, ex: loafers in gold, floral oxfords. They make amazing statement pieces for tall.

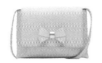

 Ruffles paired with masculine short black boots.

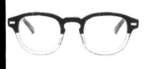

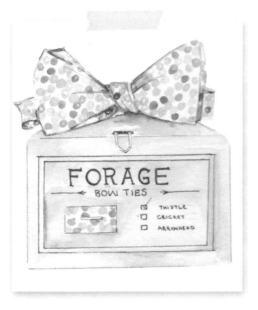

FORAGE
← BOW TIES →

☑ THISTLE
☐ CRICKET
☐ ARROWHEAD

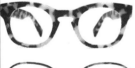

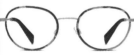

{ reflect }

· ·

· ·

· ·

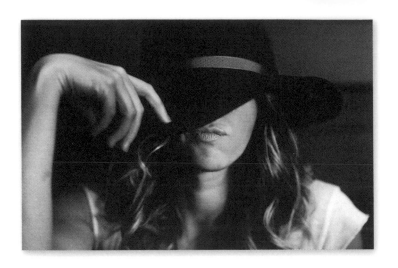

become a hat person

A wide-brimmed hat is visually pleasing on just about everyone. An angled brim can make your face seem more structured; a felted swoop holds the power to completely transform your look. Think you look weird in a hat? Chances are you're just not visually used to your image when wearing one. It's like that time you got your hair colored and swore the hairdresser was secretly out to ruin your life with the wrong shade, only to then declare it a flawless color five days later. Take this week to decide. Bring a friend along to the store for a second opinion. Plus, this challenge is a perfect one to try together.

I'm a hat fanatic (fan-hat-ic? no?) and believe that no fall wardrobe is complete without the right fedora. Here are some brims to test out.

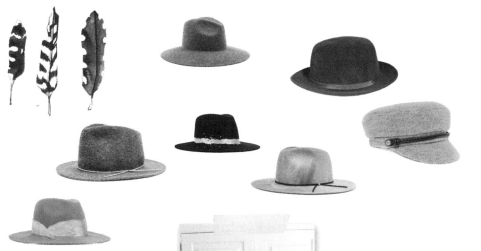

EASE IN

- Black, gray, navy.

STEP IT UP

- Maroon, olive, green, camel. A classic in an unexpected color is always a great choice.

FEELING BRAVE

- Embellishments. Grosgrain ribbon or feathers are fun and add more personality.

What's the difference between 100 likes and 1,000 likes on social media? Most likely a hat. (Don't believe me? Grab a friend and two hats, selfie, and count.)

✳ Bonus! You don't have to do much with your hair when it's under that thing.

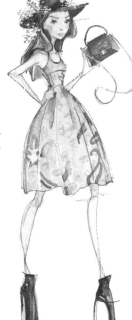

reflect

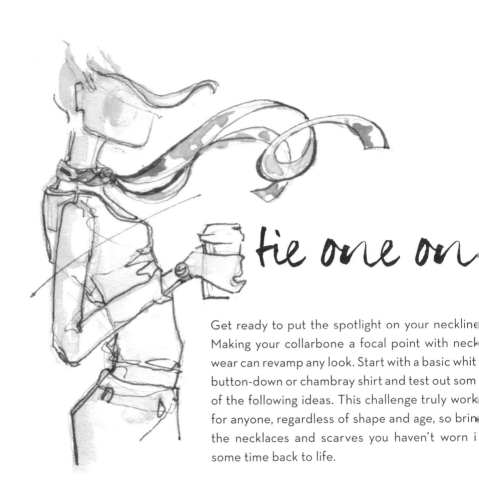

tie one on

Get ready to put the spotlight on your neckline. Making your collarbone a focal point with neck-wear can revamp any look. Start with a basic white button-down or chambray shirt and test out some of the following ideas. This challenge truly works for anyone, regardless of shape and age, so bring the necklaces and scarves you haven't worn in some time back to life.

ASE IN

Layered necklaces: Try out a few thin necklaces worn together at different lengths.

Knit scarves: Drape it and let it hang loose, or wrap it up and around you so it looks like you have a giant, thick turtleneck on.

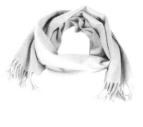
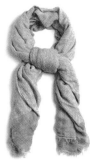

STEP IT UP

⚹ Thin silk scarves: Tied into an effortless bow, or wrapped around a few times and tied close to the neck. *oui!*

⚹ A collared shirt, buttoned all the way up, with a necklace that fits high around the neck worn just under the collar.

FEELING BRAVE

⚹ Tie-bow shirts (I adore these with a deep lip and a high waist).

⚹ Wear a bib necklace over a high neckline so it looks like part of your top.

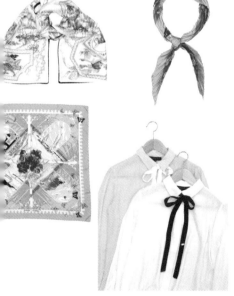

CHOKERS

Kate Moss wore one. Cinderella wore one. You're up next.

Not sure? Think of this as a short necklace. A very thin ribbon looks cool, or just pick out your favorite charm and have a chain cut into a short length for your own take on this look.

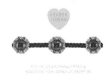

the drama!

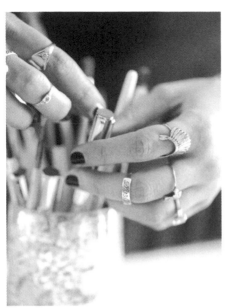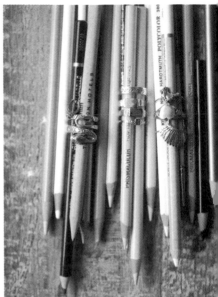

stack 'em up

You may already be a ring stacker. If you're married, you likely wear an engagement ring and a wedding band together. And single ladies are also familiar with this concept. I prefer to pile on groups of rings, mixed metals, and stones, and most end up on two fingers. Whether you plan your ring pairings or pile them on with less thought, the outcome is always different and equally cool. Plus, since everyone's jewelry collection is different, placement may be similar but no two ring stacks are alike.

What to Look For

- If you have a ring-stacking combo you are comfortable with, plan your ring purchases with that in mind.
- If you buy every ring in your ring finger size, stacking isn't an option. (Well, I guess it is—on one finger.)
- Not sure of your sizes? Walk into any ring jeweler at the mall and get sized up. It takes seconds.

How to Wear 'Em

- Keep the heaviest finger on your first hand, and bare on the second hand since it's so heavy on the other side.
- Let a very special piece stand alone on your index finger.
- Create a power stack on your middle finger.
- A thin ring next to a power stack is nice and carries the metallic across the hand.

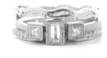

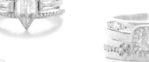

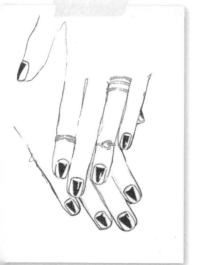

something feeling empty? add a midi ring.

✳ Make sure midis are snug. One emphatic move and they go flying across the office.

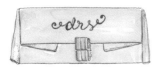

customize it

Last night I was at an event talking to a friend who said the word *monograms* with a funny snide tone in describing a recent visit to Palm Beach. This sat with me, because I kind of dig a good monogram *and Palm Beach*. I have a font obsession. I live for one-of-a-kind pieces. What's not to love?

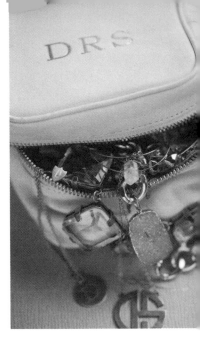

You are technically customizing all your accessories when you are choosing (or dreaming about) what color bag to invest in, cell case to put on your phone, etc. Custom and personalized pieces are my ultimate favorite option for accessories. It's time to bring them back, hard. Here are some of mine as a guide:

you don't worry about fitting in when you're custom ma[de]

MY PERSONALIZED PIECES

- Initial necklaces are cool. You can even get your child's initial (I wear my dog's initial on a signet ring).

- Name necklaces are even cooler. I wear my maiden name, which is also my grandfather's nickname, on a long gold dog tag.

- I'm a fashion illustrator and my signature is my thing, so I got it made into a literal **signature necklace**. Bonus: The messier your signature, the cooler this looks.

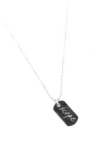

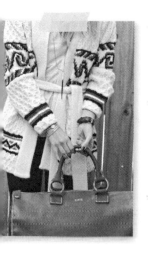

- I have a thin band bracelet that has my wedding anniversary written in roman numerals. (Love this idea for a Valentine's gift or a New Mom gift.)

- Travel gear is perfect for a stamped monogram. I have a leather travel bag with a gold mono stamp, as well as a jewelry holder with a gold zipper and monogram on top.

- A teeny-tiny pair of initial earrings: one D and one S. (I also like NY and LA for this.)

- Monograms in unexpected places. I love when my rose gold anklet with my full initials (d.r.s) peeks out from my booties.

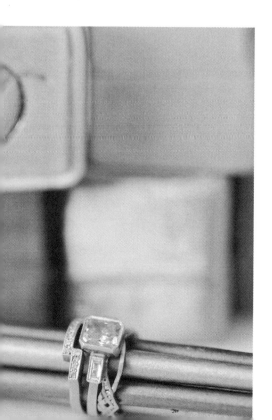

- I like the idea of friends having a word necklace (the new version of best friend necklaces).

LOBSTER

- And probably most dedicated of all my customized pieces, a stacked-band wedding ring I designed with Dawes Design. Love that I can change the bands up.

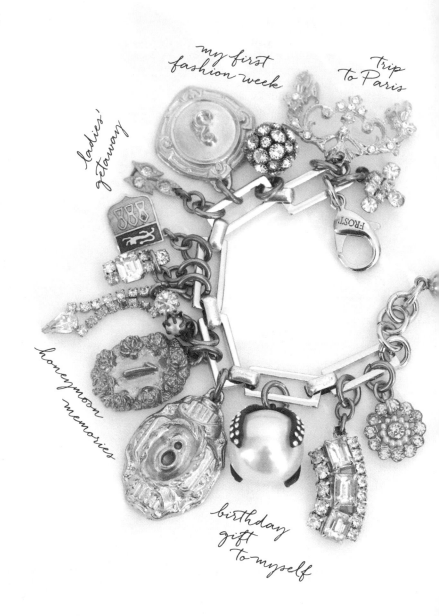

my first
fashion week

Trip
to Paris

ladies'
getaway

honeymoon
memories

birthday
gift
to myself

how charming

I cannot resist a big chunky bracelet, so I decided to bring the most personal piece of them all back into my life. Welcome back, charm bracelet. Online, I studied a few thick vintage designs I liked, and then I called my friends at Lulu Frost to bring my vision to life. Lisa, the designer, and I piled on special vintage pieces and filled spaces with traditional pieces that felt significant to me from her collection. We built a one-of-a kind beauty. Now it's your turn. Begin with one bracelet and a single charm like Lulu Frost and I did, then add charms as you collect them.

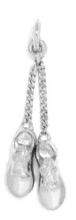

The charm doesn't have to match the occasion. I choose charms based on design alone. Choose ones you love and add them as you wish.

I think the more, the merrier, but single charms work, too.

{ reflect }

how will you get personal?

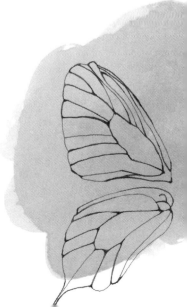

organize your bag once and for all

In the summer, I walk around with a tiny bag, or sometimes even a wristlet. Come fall, I'm filling a tote with my entire life. Without some order, I'd be digging in this bag for hours on end. Everyone's must-haves for long days are different. Grab your bag, determine what you really need to be carrying, and see how you can better organize your essentials.

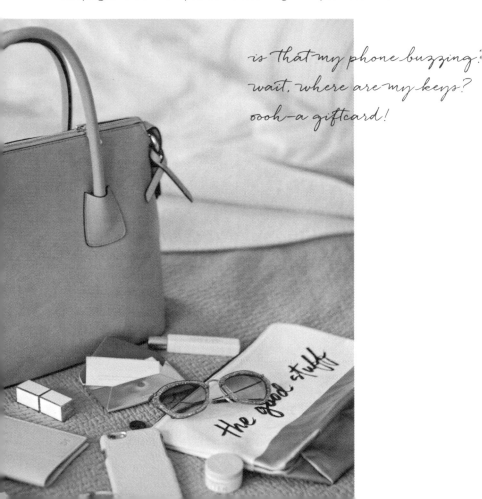

is that my phone buzzing?
wait, where are my keys?
oooh—a giftcard!

the good stuff

BEFORE:

Planner, pens, powder, makeup brushes, phone charger, wallet, keys, nail files (that I hope aren't scratching my) sunglasses, loose change, breath mints, lip glosses, soooo many receipts, Advil, perfume (please don't spill, please don't spill)...

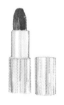 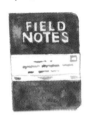  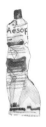 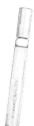

AFTER:

1. Essentials (aka "side pocket musts"). Keys, phone, wallet. Meet your new home.

2. Cord clutter cleared: Headphones and chargers get wrapped up. *life changing*.

3. Small items quarantined: I keep a smaller pretty bag inside my giant bag for those tiny items. I'm looking at you, nail files, Advil, hand sani, bobby pins, and hair ties.

4. Makeup stored safely: I keep an on-the-go makeup bag for my tweezers, small lint brush, lip balm, powder, gloss, rollerball perfume...

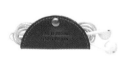 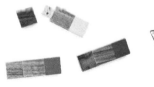

GOT TOO MANY?/GET THIS

Gift cards or receipts/A small zippered bag

Coins/A change purse

Beauty essentials/Two-for-one products like cream blush (that also works as lip color)

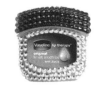

ah, it feels like a weight has been lifted off my shoulder.

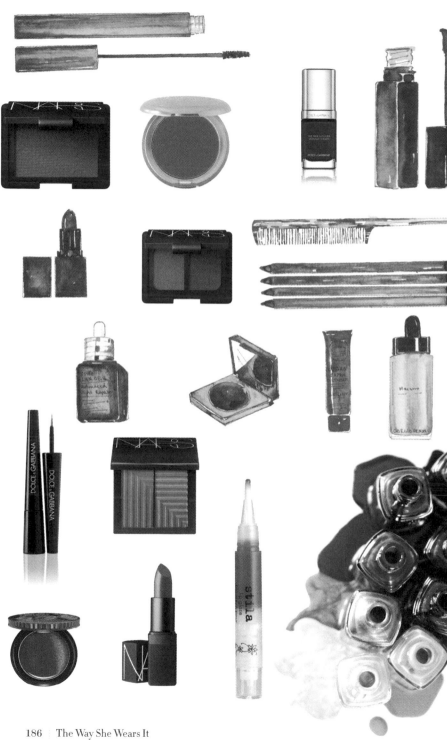

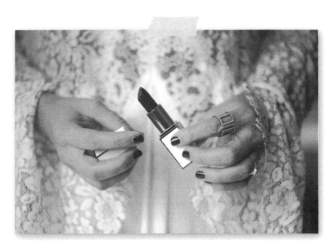

freshen up
your fall makeup bag

Every season, take a day to check in with your makeup bag. In the fall, it's out with the nude gloss and coral polish and in with matte browns and berry lipstick. Inked liner finally comes out of hibernation and makes us feel all moody again. Go hit up Sephora, make a list, grab a new eye palette (the best ones come out in the fall), and get gorgeous.

#THINGSWENEED

Strong brows	Matte everything	Dark inky liner
Cocoa shimmer	Contouring kit	Smoky eyes
Berry lips		

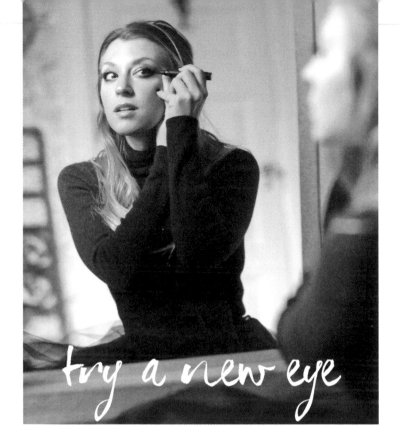

try a new eye

When heading to an event, you take extra time on your eye make-up, but on an average Wednesday, you switch back to a nude base and a quick swipe of mascara. Well, not this Wednesday. This week, choose one of the two following looks and wear them to work! Already an eyeliner pro? Give extra care to the style this time and get ready to bat those lashes at all your deadlines.

*may your coffee be hot
and your eyeliner be even.*

✳ Dust lightly with a sheer setting powder to keep your makeup in place.

FOR A CLASSIC WINGED LINER

Step 1: With a very thin ink liner, draw a small curved line from the corner of your eye outward and upward.

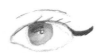

Step 2: Begin a similar line just above and connect the two at the outer end.

Step 3: From the tail end of the shape you've drawn, bring the line back in and across the top of your lid. (All the way across the eye.)

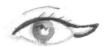

Step 4: Fill in the space at the end.

✳ An ink liner is classic and will give you a nice crisp line. Beginners: Keep the line thin at first and then thicken it for more drama.

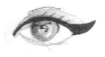

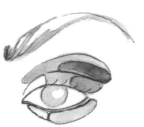

FOR THE PERFECT SMOKY EYE

You'll need three shades: light, medium, and dark. For a brown smoky eye, go with taupe, caramel, and dark brown. For a traditional black smoky eye, go with light gray, medium gray, and black.

Step 1: Use the light color all over your eyelid and in the crease. Line the bottom eyelid in this shade.

Step 2: Add the mid shade to the middle of your eyelid and in the crease, and then to the middle under the eye.

Step 3: Add the darkest shade to the outer corner of your eye and in the corner of the crease. Blend.

✳ Enhance with an eyeliner (creamy pencil, not ink) that's rich in pigment. A deep brown or eggplant for a brown smoky eye, or black for a traditional smoky eye.

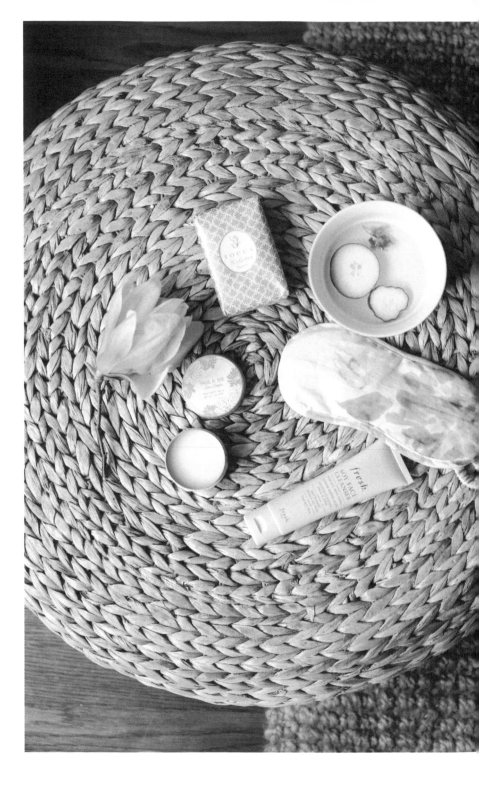

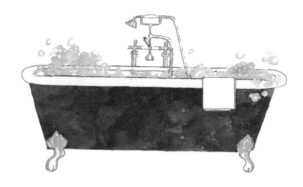

the challenge continues . . .

GET A SPRAY TAN

"But Dallas, the summer's over—"

I know. That's the point. Sometimes you just need a little glow. Don't worry about looking like the cast of *Jersey Shore*—new spray services will customize your shade.

GET MINDFUL ABOUT YOUR HAIR

Luxury shampoo makes your washing routine a little more alluring. My favorite is currently Kérastase. While you're at it, grab a hair treatment mask and schedule yourself (yes, in your planner) for a weekly or bi-weekly at-home treatment. I use Fekkai's biweekly and I am hooked, not just on the product but on the entire process. It's my version of mindfulness.

TRY A DARK MANI OR LIPPY

Fall marks the return of dark lips and polishes. Try a glossy navy nail or a deep brown lip. (But wearing both together might have you feeling like a vampire so leave that combo for the runway.)

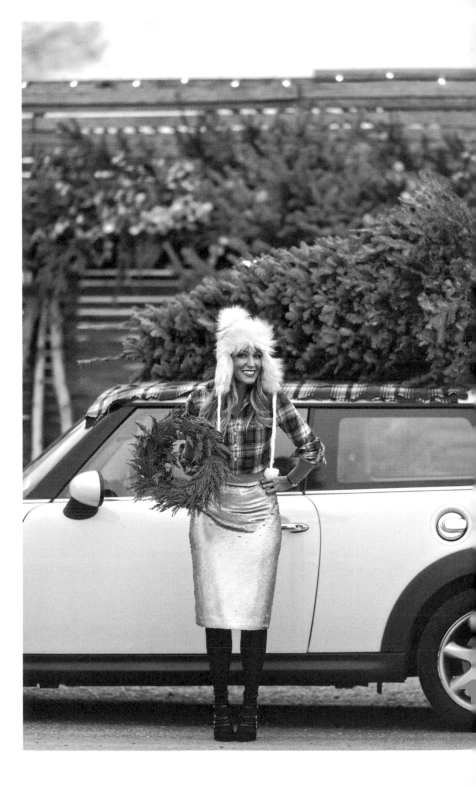

WINTER

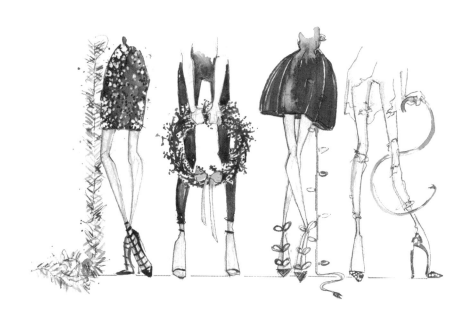

Months of cabin-inspired menswear. The warmth of the first snowfall. And my personal favorite: justifiable hibernation.

I get it—it's cold. There are short days, long nights, and brutally low temps.

But there are also big coats and bonfires. And carbs are part of your diet again—weeeee!

I know wintertime complaints are second nature, but stop being a hater and start enjoying these next few months of humidity-free hair. You're about to embark on a season that begins with tinsel and ends in complete cashmere coziness.

'Tis the season to see and be seen. Holiday parties are back on the calendar, and you get to amp up your glam factor for months, not just on New Year's Eve. Speaking of which, it's the perfect time to refocus your style resolutions. Challenge yourself even more this season by trying new looks and making the time for yourself that you deserve. Those new shoes you bought for yourself while gift shopping will be a killer kick start.

This season is pure magic. Dogs wear sweaters! Your winter goal is to hold on to the wonder past December. I know … those twinkle lights really help.

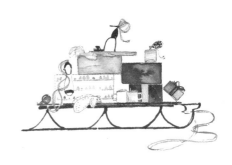

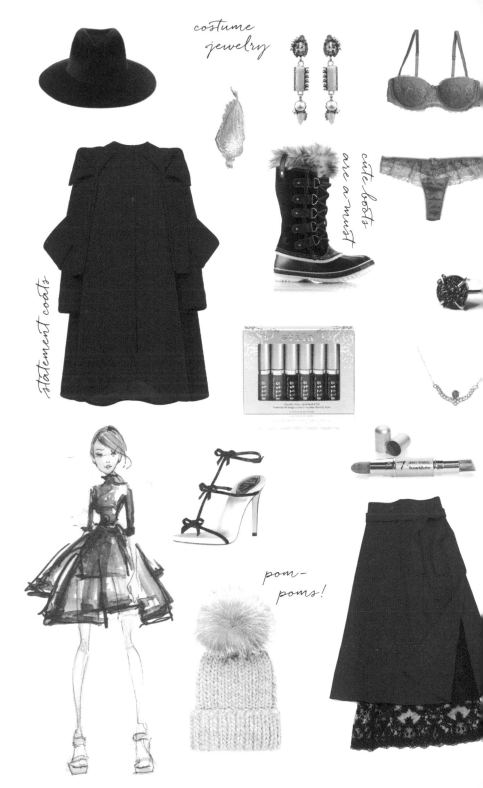

costume
jewelry

cute boots
are a must

statement coats

pom-
poms!

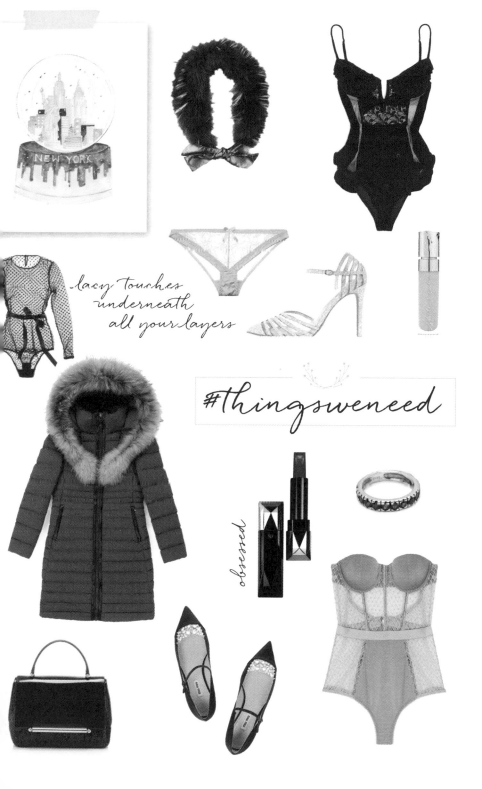

lacy touches
underneath
all your layers

#thingsweneed

obsessed

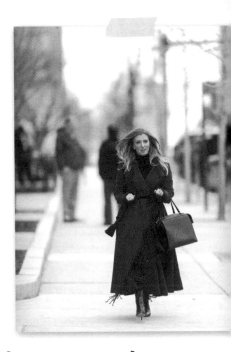

it's what's on the outside that counts

The scene: New York Fashion Week 2013. We arrived bright eyed with barely liftable luggage, filled to the brim with sky-high stilettos and the best dresses of the season.

And then a blizzard hit.

(but . . . but, my shoes?)

The shows must go on, so we headed to the NYFW tents in the whiteout. Somehow everyone still looked impeccable, cloaked in delicately woven hand-knit hats in rich hues, fitted ladylike coats, and long leather gloves. We all could have been in our pajamas underneath this outerwear and it wouldn't have mattered, because on the coldest days of winter, it doesn't really matter what's underneath after all.

Today, think about your outerwear look as your outfit. There are four parts to this challenge:

1. Your coat—this will have the biggest impact on your winter wardrobe. Forget about the black bubble jacket: there is nothing that will make you feel less chic than dressing like the Michelin Man. Find a coat in

a color and fit that makes you feel good. Whether it's an expensive-feeling wool wrap or a belted A-line, look for something more polished than your usual choice.

2. A bag that complements your outerwear. If you choose a structured coat, choose a structured bag.

✱ The slimmer or more fitted the coat, the more accessories you can add without adding volume.

3. A pair of boots that suits your style as well as your coat choice, and that you can walk in when it gets icy. It's winter!

4. One winter accessory staple: scarf, gloves, hat, snood, sunglasses (baby, it's bright outside).

Rethink and pair these four items that you already own to complete the challenge and remain put-together for the rest of the season. When you get bored with this look, remember that different accessories can completely change the look of your coat, and switch up the combination.

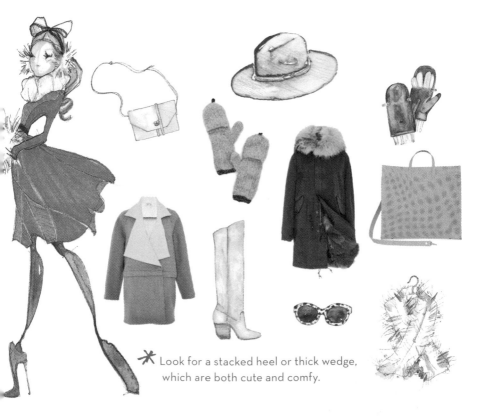

✱ Look for a stacked heel or thick wedge, which are both cute and comfy.

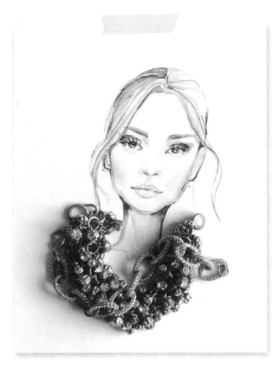

 I can't resist a statement piece. My personal collection includes a large brass floral bracelet and a vintage Chanel medallion.

make a statement

Today you'll pick one ornate accessory and let it do all the talking. Statement pieces can come in all shapes and sizes. If it's unique and eye-catching, this is your piece. These accessories can take any casual article of clothing to the next level. Keep in mind that "statement" doesn't have to mean oversized. Go for something just out of your comfort zone.

STATEMENT EARRINGS

EASE IN

- Small sparklers with gray tees.

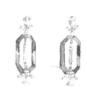

STEP IT UP

- Pair your crystals with army coats.

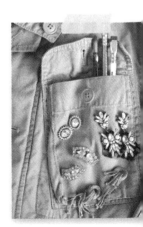

FEELING BRAVE

- Statement drop earrings with a tee and a silk scarf.

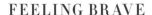 For drop earrings, the higher the
neckline, the longer the drop. The
lower the neckline, the shorter the
drop.

STATEMENT NECKLACE

EASE IN

- With all black for some edge.
- With a T-shirt and a pony.

STEP IT UP

- With a striped button-down shirt
  (roll the sleeves and mess up the
  collar and voilà).
- Stacked on top of one another—double up!

FEELING BRAVE

- With a sweatshirt and blazer.
- Wear over a high, already embellished neckline.

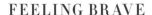 Keep an extra statement necklace at work. Throw it on last
minute to feel more put together when an unexpected meeting turns up
on the calendar.

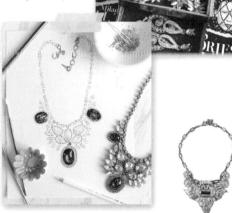

MORE STATEMENTS WAITING TO BE MADE

- A large gold and pearl cuff with a crew neck sweater and
  boyfriend jeans.
- Statement shoes worn with prints.

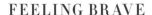 Pair your bling with something else sparkly
for maximum impact. { crystal earrings ×
embellished pencil skirt }

- Ballet-inspired wrap sweaters
- Silk tanks and shorts
- Gray joggers
- Candles
- Leg warmers or loose-fitting over-the-knee socks
- A cashmere or soft scarf
- Silk sleep masks

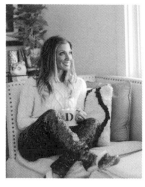

I shop dancewear sites for dusty-pink wrap sweaters and fuzzy leg warmers. Then I scour yoga sites for black leggings that hit mid-foot.

here's to the ladies who lounge

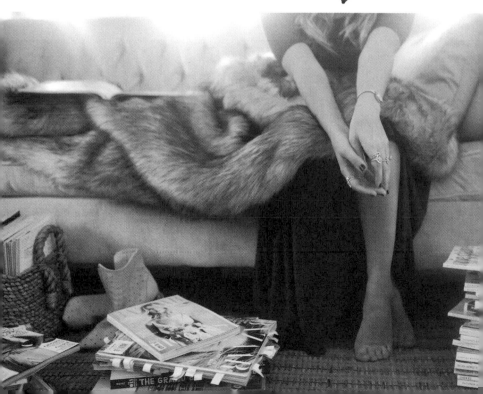

{ pj's all day }

Hooray for a snow day! You've been dreaming about this day for so long that you've even made a checklist.

WHAT YOU WANT TO DO:

Wake up before your alarm, listen to relaxing music, do some morning stretches, make a tea with the sunrise (wait, I don't even drink tea), meditate, try an A.M. face mask, reflect and journal, cozy up with Hemingway by the fireplace, eat a healthy lunch, nap with the pups, watch a movie in bed, light some candles, stay away from your phone and e-mail for an entire day . . .

WHAT YOU DO:

Wake up.

Schlep around in your pajamas all day with your phone attached to your hand. *womp.*

It's time to get rid of your stretched-out sweats. Beautiful loungewear will take your lazy days to luxurious.

you're getting verrry sleeeepy.

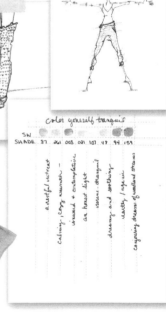

* I fold my loungewear neatly and keep it placed near a lavender linen drawer sachet, so when I put it on I'm already halfway to deep relaxation. Om . . .

Soft colors = Soft emotions

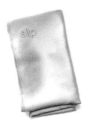

GANGSTA NAPPER

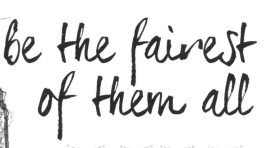

be the fairest of them all

Fair Isle: Named after a tiny island in the north of Scotland, this is a form of colorwork knitting characterized by bands of multicolored geometric patterns. See also: Dallas's winter obsessions.

As an artist, I'm naturally drawn to multicolored garments—which is why I love Fair Isle knits. Every time I wear one, I can feel all my Scandinavian ski lodge dreams coming true. Fair Isle makes for an easy-to-wear stand-alone piece since the mixed shades make a little statement. It's time to embrace these cozy decorative patterns and get some Fair Isle street style.

Psst: Shop the men's section for the best selection. You're welcome.

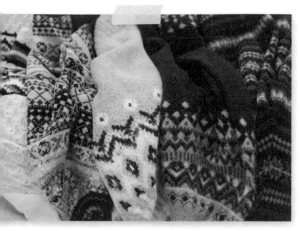

* Easy add-on for every
level: camp socks.

HOW TO STYLE YOUR FAVORITE FAIR ISLE KNIT

EASE IN

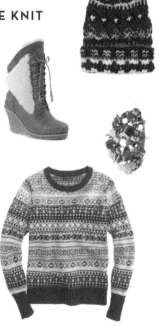

- Try it with dark denim, brown booties, rhinestones, and a small touch of Sherpa to really play up its cold characteristics.
- Pair a more fitted sweater with men's trousers for some sophistication.
- A cardigan-style sweater worn over a flannel and ripped jeans.
- A classic-cut sweater, a big belt, and a blingy ring.

STEP IT UP

- A belted Fair Isle wrap sweater worn with a wide-brimmed hat.
- With a denim midi skirt and booties, or a wide-leg pant for a '70s vibe.
- Worn with a plaid scarf.

FEELING BRAVE

- Under a furry jacket (takes you from snow bunny to bombshell).
- Under a blazer for a vest-like feeling.
- Embellished, for the win.

get fitted and knitted

Cable knit is classic. So classic, in fact, that it can sometimes feel very, well, let's be honest, uptight. When I say cable knit, you think more about country clubs than of high fashion. Even so, it's a staple most of us own. This challenge is not your grandmother's cable knit. (You don't want to pair cable knit with anything too proper.) Today, we'll make crochet cool again by owning these threads and putting your own twist on your knits.

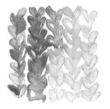

cable knit
× fireplaces
× hot cocoa

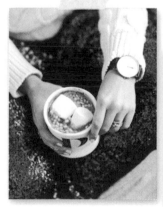

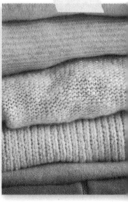

lumbersexual:
the affinity for bearded
men in knitted things.

EASE IN

- Turtleneck cable knit x skinny jeans x black pointy-toe booties x a bun.
- Go oversized and pair with leather leggings.
- Undo your hair. A messy pony or loose waves add a carefree touch.

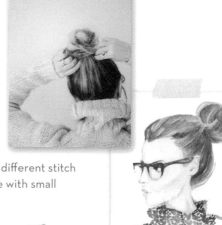

✴ When shopping for cable knit, keep an eye open for something unique, a different stitch or an unexpected color. I prefer mine with small knit poms sprinkled throughout.

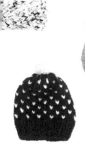
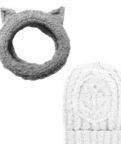
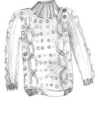

STEP IT UP

- A cable-knit cardigan with a T-shirt and flat no-lace booties for a laid-back vibe.
- Cable-knit slouchy beanie and mittens paired with aviators. *over a thin sweater. sans jacket. plus coffee.*
- Tuck it into front-pleated trousers and add mirrored shades.

FEELING BRAVE

- Tuck it into a maxi skirt for a touch of glam that's surprisingly easy to pull off.
- With sequined pants and heels for a real moment.
- Bring it out of season. Over a sundress or denim shorts on the beach at dusk is my personal favorite.

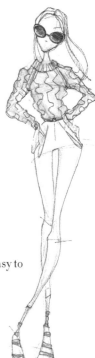

tuxedo jackets × sneaks

High ponies and shades make this look extra cool.

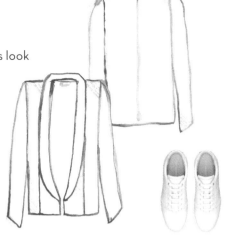

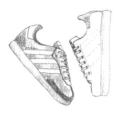

ballet slippers × cozy sweaters

Ballet slippers are my version of house slippers.

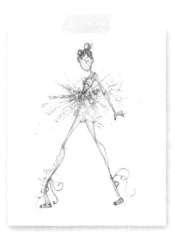

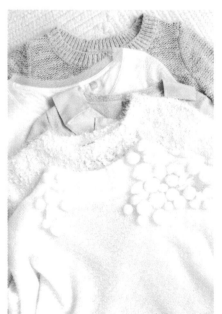

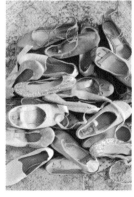

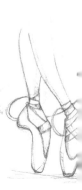

perfect pairings

we go together like:

{ *leather* × *gingham* }

You can even add oxfords here for extra points.

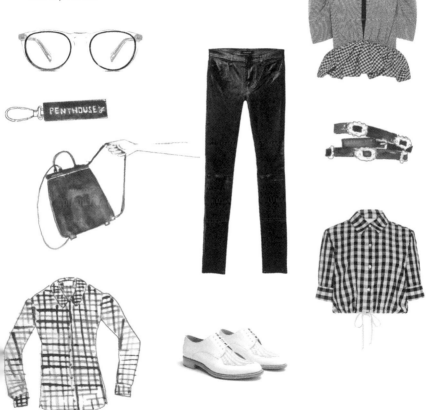

Design Your Winter Palette

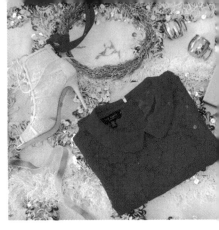

When the first snowflake falls (sqeeee), I throw on some comfy clothes, hit the record player with holiday pop music, and race to the closet to begin my plan. I like my winter full of dramatic deep tones and woolen frosty pastels. I reach for the more inspirational pieces I've collected over the years: silky emerald pants, rich scarlet dresses, and shimmery navy lace. I'm inspired by the seriousness of those colors against the bleached snow-lined streets.

A contrast of gentle pastels begins to take over my armoire. Fuzzy winter whites, fawns, and dusty-pink knitwear appears in proud, neatly folded stacks on my shelves. I take a step back, and once I feel confident that I'm primed for spontaneous snow angels, I add metallics. Glistening gold detailing and snowy silver embellishments as accents, a flurry of excitement about the approaching season, and a little shopping list, of course.

Let's create your winter color story. Place your notes or inspiration here:

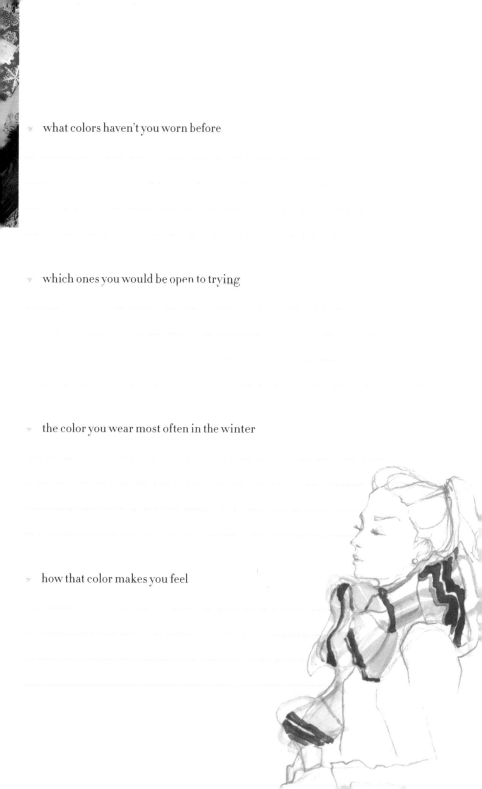

- what colors haven't you worn before

- which ones you would be open to trying

- the color you wear most often in the winter

- how that color makes you feel

have a monochromatic moment

So far in this book, we've been playing with unusual pairings that produce unexpected wins, so this challenge may feel a bit unnatural if it's something you haven't tried before. The challenge is to wear one color from head to toe. You're likely to have gravitated toward a color in the past, so head to your closet and see if you have a bag, pants, a top, and heels in the same shade. Put all those items on together and see if it works. You may have to play with your pairings a bit, but when the combination is just right, you'll know it.

✳ Have a long solid dress? That counts, too. Look for a matching bag and shoe.

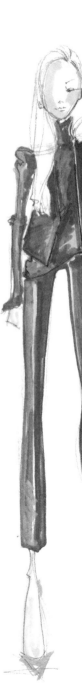

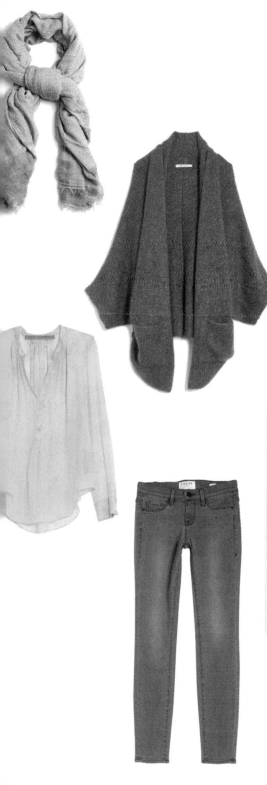

EASE IN

- Start with the basics: black, navy, gray.

STEP IT UP

- Taupe, emerald green, deep berry.

FEELING BRAVE

- Poppy red, mustard yellow

Head-to-toe caramel is my world.

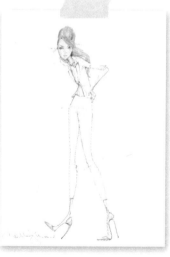

wear black and navy

In order to keep my relationship with my grandmother strong, you should probably not discuss this next challenge with her. She is one of the many people who have grown up believing that wearing black and navy together is quite possibly the biggest fashion faux pas you can commit. Not true! I've done some color research and discovered the single reason people think that black and navy paired together looks bad: The colors are so similar, it can easily look like you accidentally wore navy when you thought it was black in the darkness of your morning routine. The key to avoiding that misstep? Focusing on differences in color and texture.

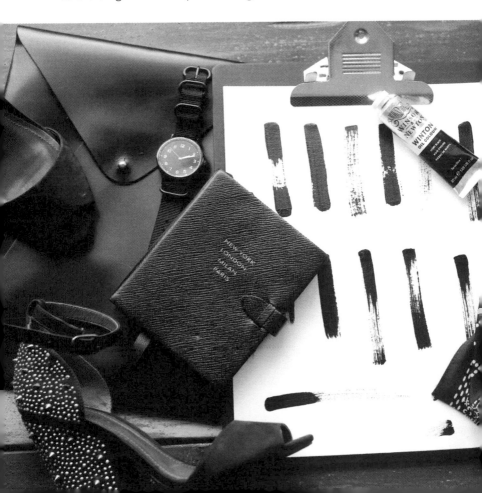

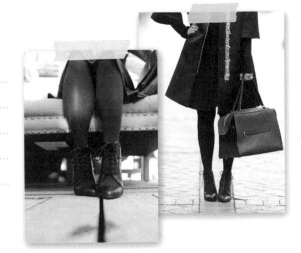

*your dark jeans
don't count as
avy. sorry, sista.)*

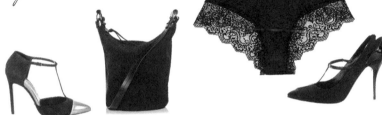

> This challenge is a well-loved trick of some of the wealthiest
> and most polished women I know. Try it with an open mind
> and see for yourself. When paired correctly, the colors look
> expensive, and often very French.

There are countless pairing options here, so I'll just get you
started...

- Black skirt x navy silk blouse.
- Navy dress x black booties x bare legs.
- Navy dress x thin black belt.
- All black x navy eyeshadow... *heyyyy now.*

Get started on this challenge in three steps!

1. List all the black items of clothing you own.
2. List all the navy items of clothing you own.
3. Mix up the lists.

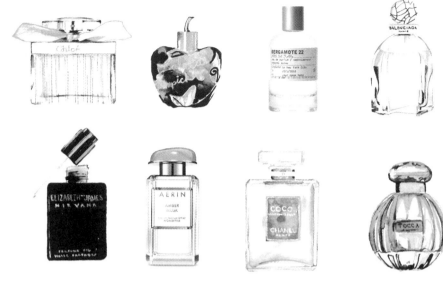

what's your scent story?

You're never fully dressed without ~~a smile~~ *Chanel no.5.*

Years ago, someone told me that French women wear perfume every day. They continued, "A signature scent is an essential part of their everyday routine, and they simply wouldn't think about walking out the door without a spritz of perfume." Was that true? I didn't care—what a beautiful idea it was! It was then that I began my scent collection, and this page is where you'll begin yours.

Scent can evoke the strongest of memories. **Lolita Lempicka** reminds me of my first trip to New York Fashion Week when everything seemed like a whirlwind of new experiences. I swear to this day I think I smell this every time a model stomps by me. **Burberry London** reminds me of my wedding, since my husband somehow snuck away into a store on a vacation and I was so moved by the sneaky gesture that I saved it to wear until my wedding day. **Elizabeth and James Nirvana Black** will always remind me of the full day of publisher meetings I went to as I pitched this very book. I asked around and the sweet story continues:

"Growing up my best friends were Grass and Heaven. I was a Dream girl myself. None of us could pull off Om, but we all wanted to."

Comme des Garçons reminds one of my bests of her triumphant return to life after a breakup, **Cherry Blossom** scents remind my mom of the holiday season, and I have a friend who swears by a very popular pop singer's scent—but tells people it's **Miss Dior** when they ask. Everyone has a scent story. What's yours?

How do you find your signature scent(s)? Spray. Wear. Repeat.

You may already have a signature scent, but I invite you to expand your collection. I like to keep all the sparkling bottles on display on a vintage mirrored tray just like my grandmother did. After I'm dressed every morning, I visit my collection and decide what scent I'm feeling like for the day ahead. Am I in a sweet mood (Viktor and Rolf Flowerbomb) or do I need a strong state of mind for this meeting (Tom Ford Noir)?

* For the holidays, tell your family you could use some perfume, and leave the scent up to them. I give people perfume as gifts all the time to force them to try something new and maybe be responsible for a new scent story.

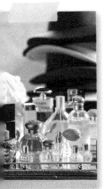

"i've never met an atomizer i didn't like."

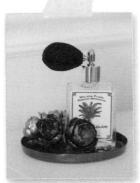

#THINGSWENEED

1. Something special to display your collection on. A vintage sterling tray, a mirrored vanity tray, or get creative with a large platter like this one trimmed in gold.
2. Beautiful bottles. You are creating a curated collection here. Most perfumes have multiple bottle designs for the same fragrance. Choose the one that's most "you."
3. Advanced collectors can add vintage perfume bottles, rollers, and atomizers into that mix.

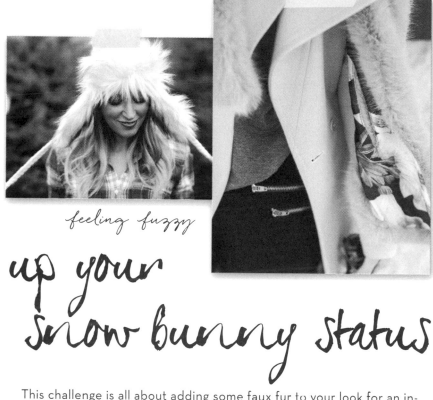

feeling fuzzy

up your snow bunny status

This challenge is all about adding some faux fur to your look for an instant style update. No need to get into the fur controversy since there are so many amazing faux-fur options. A little bit of faux fur goes a long way in your winter wardrobe, and these days your options are endless. Everyone from Ted Baker to Rachel Zoe have been paying extra attention to making sure their faux options are just the right amount of soft so that you can try this trend while remaining animal friendly. What is it about fur? By adding a single piece, you're not only adding an additional layer, but also another texture and sometimes even color to your look.

EASE IN

- Go for items that are removable—a long faux-fur scarf is effortless.
- A knit hat with a small faux-fur topper is a simple start.

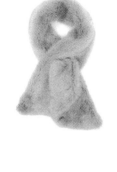

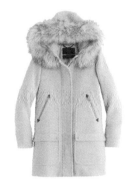

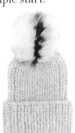

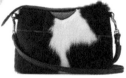

STEP IT UP

- Try a cropped faux-fur jacket paired with tailored pants.
- A faux-fur vest worn belted over a turtleneck.
- A faux-fur trapper hat is fun and perfect for all holiday adventures.

FEELING BRAVE

- Try your faux fur in a color—better yet, try a color that matches your coat. *gray! emerald! oxblood!*

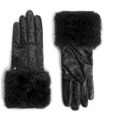

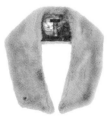

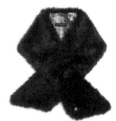

✳ Shop bridal sites for amazing and often custom faux-fur stoles.

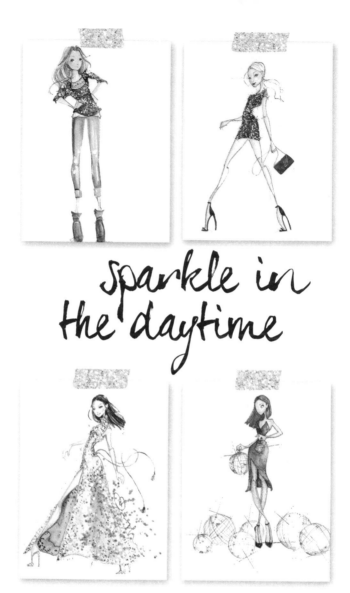

sparkle in the daytime

Winter is the season for sparkle. Therefore, it's the season *to* sparkle. While I wholeheartedly believe you should pile on the shine year-round, many ladies like to keep the sequins to the evening of December 31. Everyone knows how to wear sequins at night: To a party. On a dress. Tough stuff. So for this challenge, we are mastering something a bit more difficult: sequins in the daylight. You can do it, and I'm going to show you how.

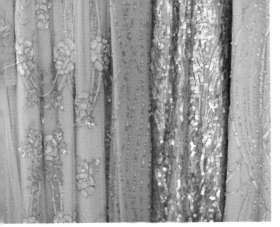

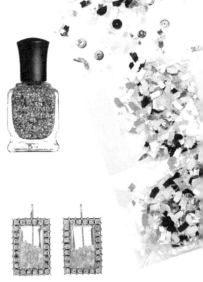

ASE IN

Glittery/embellished flats, a clutch, or a glitter
pedicure.
Sequin-embellished cardigan over a T-shirt with jeans
and flats.

 I prefer my sequins paired with
something casual. Loose jeans,
sneaks, and a minimal men's watch.

TEP IT UP

Sequined pencil skirt and flannel shirt.
Long sequined maxi skirt and loose T-shirt. I like
Chucks here, too.

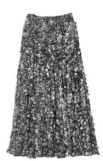

quins shimmer best
hen your makeup is
esh and light.

FEELING BRAVE

- Sequined pants and a crewneck sweater is an
  unexpected pairing.
- Try a sequined long-sleeved top with tailored pants
  for a more sophisticated getup.

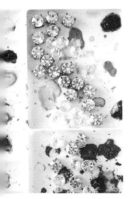

be a bag lady

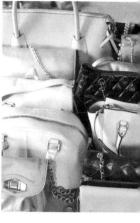

Your bag is always with you, and should not be overlooked, big or small. I have a friend who always has the right bag. Every time she stops over, I notice and comment on her purse. She's naturally gifted in bag selection, so for this challenge I went straight to the source to uncover the top five bags you need in your collection:

1. BLACK "NIGHT-OUT" BAG

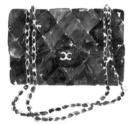

The above mentioned friend calls this her "bar-night purse," which makes complete sense. I'm always sitting across from her with my giant bag on my lap because I don't want to place it on the floor, while she is hands-free.

A small black purse with a strap, not necessarily worn as a cross-body but always with a strap, will make sure you are ready to cheers at any moment. All it needs to fit are your phone, thin wallet, keys, and lipstick.

You can't go wrong with pebbled black leather or anything with an exposed gold zipper. Special detail like tassles or unique zipp placement are even bette

2. A LARGER STYLE IN BROWN OR GRAY

This is your "everyday" bag. Think dinner with the ladies and running midday errands.

Try a gray—it's unique and plays nice with dark color pastels. (Yes, you can wea pastels in winter.)

It's bigger than your bar-night bag, because you want to be able to tote around a camera, book, planner, *Sour Patch Kids, you know—necessities.*

A satchel or hobo is nice here because of the sizing, and ideally you'll want some-

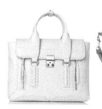

thing that has top handles and also has a
long strap for when your hands are full*of*
shopping bags.

 I like cream, winter white, and
sometimes very light dusty-
pink shades.

3. A STRUCTURED LARGE BAG FOR WORK

This is the bag that makes me feel like a powerhouse
in meetings. When I walk into a room and place my
bag on the table, I feel like it's nodding at the other
members like "yeah, that's right." I especially like a
structured bag in the wintertime; it streamlines everything
when scarves and layers pile up (otherwise, you truly look
like a bag lady).

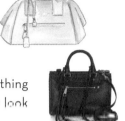

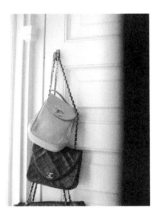

4. WILDCARD/COLLECTOR BAG

Sometimes you see a bag you just have to have,
regardless of its practicality. If you love it, you
should have it. Just make sure you have practi-
cal options in addition to this knockout.

 I like my wildcard bags to be just that, bold and
brave in color combo. When I invest in a designer
bag, I lean toward a purse that has a number of
shades within. It almost always complements at
least one shade I have on. Sometimes, the less it
matches, the more it works.

5. A LARGE TOTE

For everything else in life.

✳ A classic leather tote in a deep color
like black or raisin is a wise addition and
will be a forever part of your wardrobe.
Absolutely timeless.

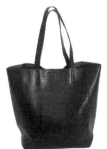

Ready to start your collection?

*Go directly to Rebecca Minkoff
or Elizabeth and James.
Do not pass Go.
Do not collect $200.*

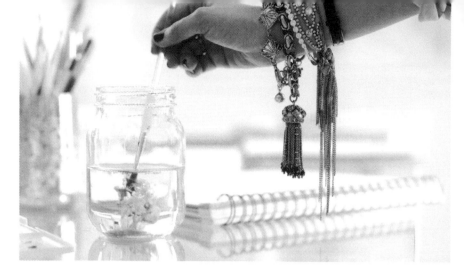

stay golden

How could I possibly write a book urging you to embrace the luxury in every day and not include the color of luxury? Quick word association: When I say "gold," what words come to mind?

*Rich Powerful Expensive Treasure Extravagance Confident
Glowing Warm*

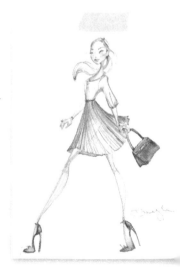

Today I'll encourage you to add (pile on, whatever) gold jewelry and accessories for an immediate glam factor, and then reflect on how wearing your favorite gold pieces makes you feel.

a little luxury never hurt nobody

Gold channels masculine energy and is associated with the power of the sun, compared to silver, which is associated with feminine energy and the sensitivity of the moon. Get ready to feel strong. Gold illuminates and enhances the items directly around it.

EASE IN

- Focus on the hands. Minimum two pieces of gold jewelry per hand, paired with a deep, rich, glossy shade of nail polish like navy or chocolate.
- A bag with gold detailing paired with a simple turtleneck and denim.

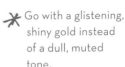

Go with a glistening, shiny gold instead of a dull, muted tone.

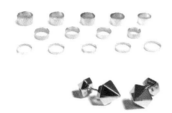

STEP IT UP

- Gold metallic flats with ankle-length denim.
- Gold aviators in the winter look shockingly cool with your fitted coat.

Have an old coat you're bored with? Switch out the buttons to gold ones for a quick update.

FEELING BRAVE

- Gold heels with your work pants and top feels so festive. I like mine with a bright poppy-orange lip.
- If you can find one, a metallic maxi skirt is the ultimate statement piece.

 reflect }

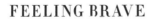

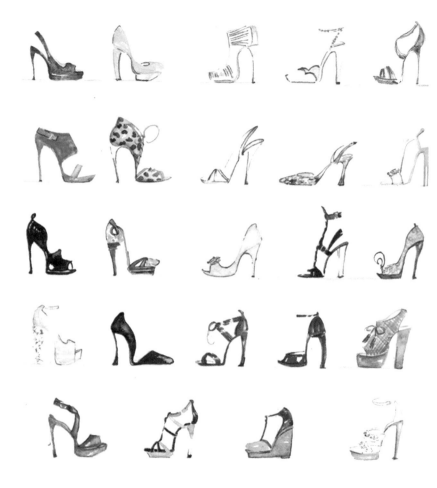

begin plotting your ultimate shoe collection

Unless you live in the tropics (*I wiiiish*), shoes are a crucial part of every wardrobe. They complete your look and allow you to make a quick getaway if the party isn't where it's at. It's important to have just the right shoe to make an impact, so I'm all for building an extensive shoe wardrobe. Before you begin, I'll need you to take a little inventory to break out of your current shoe rut.

Chances are you are buying the same shoe in the same styles every season without even realizing it. Today you are going to take inventory, and take some serious note of what you are buying. The goal is to decide what you can get rid of, what you don't need another pair of, and (best part) what you can add to the collection.

Go to your shoe storage with a notepad and a pen. You'll begin a shoe type list.

Pull out a pair of boots? Write "boots" and place said boot in a boot pile.

Next pair: Leather flip-flops? Add "flip flops" to your category list and start a new pile for flip-flops only.

Continue until you have a full list of shoe types and you're surrounded by little piles of shoes. Your list might look something like this: *Wedges, Over-the-Knee Boots, Sandals, Booties, Peep-toes, T-straps,* and *Flats.*

Look at each pile and list the number you have in each category.

If you have 3 wedges, 1 over-the-knee boot, 5 sneakers, and 875,374 flats—then you're going to take a break from flats for a while. Say it out loud if you need to.

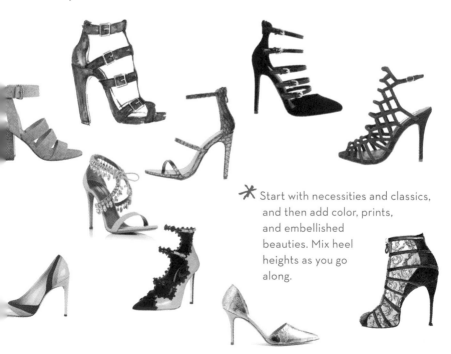

✱ Start with necessities and classics, and then add color, prints, and embellished beauties. Mix heel heights as you go along.

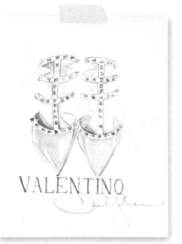

VALENTINO

Also, pay attention to color patterns here. If you have six pair of black flats, the next color you bring home will be nude or neon or nothing, you hear me? If you have four or more of the same color shoes in the same pile, do you know what else you have? Too many. Let one go.

You did an amazing job today! Treat yourself to ONE new pair of shoes, as long as they are a new style or color. Or both.

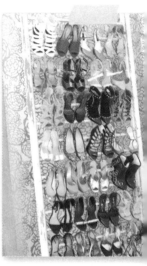

i hang my heels from a piece of an old window i found at a salvage shop and pile my flats in vintage metal bin stacks. get creative with your shoe storage.

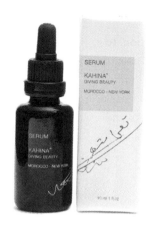

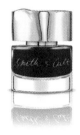

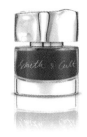

#THINGSWENEED

Red lips
Strong liner
Matte skin
A deep, sleek side part

Icy tones
Navy nails
Creamy lotion

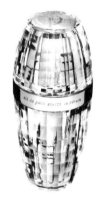

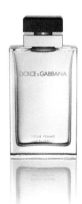

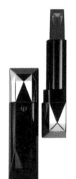

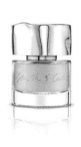

freshen up your winter makeup bag

Let the sparkling palettes in every window be your inspiration right now. Even if just for these few months, glam up your bag with two to three metallics and dark shades. A pewter shadow here, a deep brown liquid liner there. Along with a brick-brown lip, and a neutral matte blush these little additions will have you feeling refined and sophisticated.

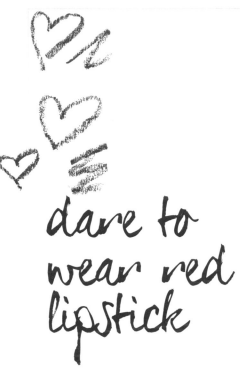

dare to wear red lipstick

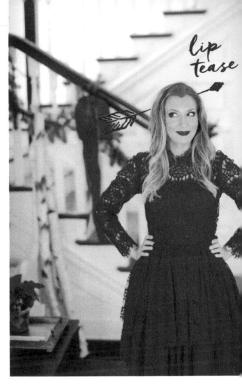

lip tease

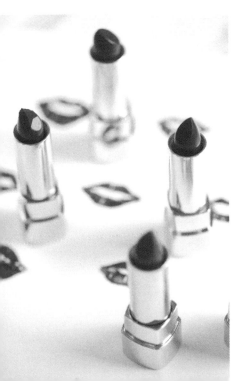

A red lip is the beginner's guide to looking like an instant expert, so be prepared to make a big jump today. Red lipstick is a state of mind. Find your shade and get ready to take care of business. You'll need some extra confidence to pull this off. Take a deep breath and have some faith in yourself—you *can* own this look.

* Very little eye makeup today, ladies.

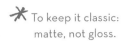

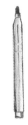

#THINGSWENEED

Lip brush
Lip exfoliator
Liner (red or nude)

Lipstick
Makeup remover, cotton
pads (trust me on this)

To keep it classic:
matte, not gloss.

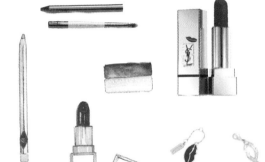

a kiss in the air and a skip in your step.

EASE IN

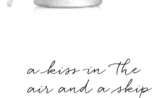

⚡ Look for a sheer formula.

STEP IT UP

⚡ A creamier version with brown tones.

FEELING BRAVE

⚡ A bright poppy. My fave? Stila Stay All Day red.

Please check all that apply:

Confidence boost ___
Assertive _ _ _
Powerful ___
Mood boost ___

Psst: Your mouth is a focal point, so don't forget the finger test to keep your lipstick off your teeth.

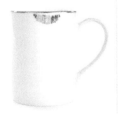

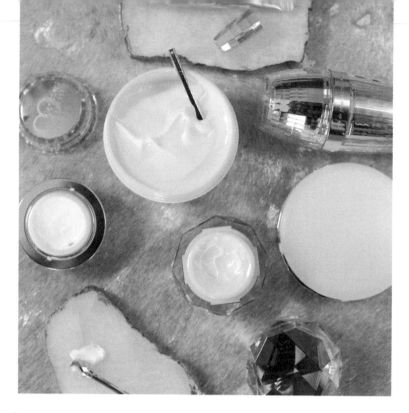

freshen up your foundation

There hits a point at the end of January every year when your skin starts feeling extra levels of b l a h. You can't remember the last time you've seen the sun, and the weather conditions seem to be taking a toll on your skin type. Dry skin, dry lips, uneven skin tone, breakouts—each of my friends has a different "symptom" that alerts them to this moment. A little bit of extra attention and a seasonal change-up of product is the ultimate cure for when you can't

✳ Ask questions, and try in-store ON your face. Hey! I see you. Your hand is NOT your face.

get to St. Barts. Your skin is a different shade in the wintertime, so simply changing out the shades of your product can bring back its luminosity.

Step 1: Switch from your regular daily lotion to one with a creamier consistency. Don't ignore your neck and lips.

✳ Don't be afraid to try a pricier new product. Choose a store with a return policy that allows you to exchange in case you get the shade wrong the first time.

Step 2: While the light is natural, get thee to a cosmetics store and focus your attention toward face makeup only: foundation, primer, concealer, spot touch-up. Stay focused in the cosmetics store—no new blushes, don't get distracted by the sparkling palettes—the base is what's important here.

Step 3: To get the color just right, apply it in natural light or use a magnifying mirror. Double check that jawline and blend, blend, blend.

When your skin looks this good, you can shine in a simple sweater, so don't overlook getting this shade right. Test out your fresh face with a solid sweater, denim, booties, and not much else to see just how confident your glowing skin can make you feel.

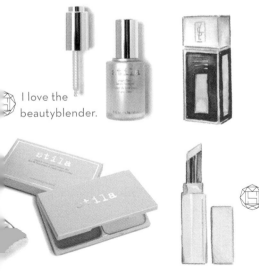

I love the beautyblender.

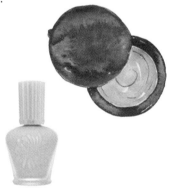

Garnier BB Cream is my go-to foundation. Often hidden in the hair section with the rest of their products instead of the traditional cosmetics section of the drugstore, it doesn't disappoint.

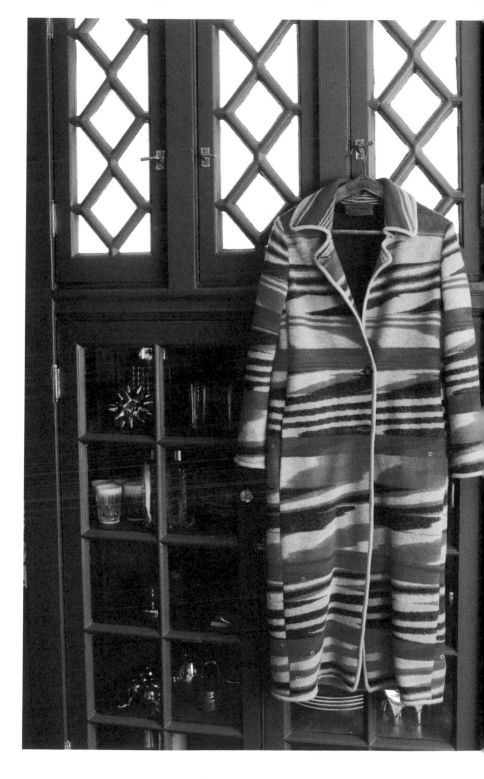

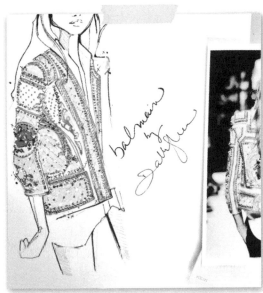

the challenge continues . . .

ADD A TOUCH OF VELVET

There's nothing more lush than velvet, and there's no better time to wear it. A top with a touch of velvet, or a crushed velvet dresswill work for every holiday fete. I also LOVE a velvet heel.

GO LONG

Enter your next holiday party with an amazing statement coat. Go with a print or a deep rich shade, and go long. Any ankle-length coat sweeping across the room is dramatic and majestic.

SEARCH FOR A FANCY CLUTCH

Look for an embellished clutch, keeping an eye out for rhinestones, ribbons, and statement buckles. Tote it for the season (whether you are dressed up or not), and then bring it back out later in the year to update your favorite LBD.

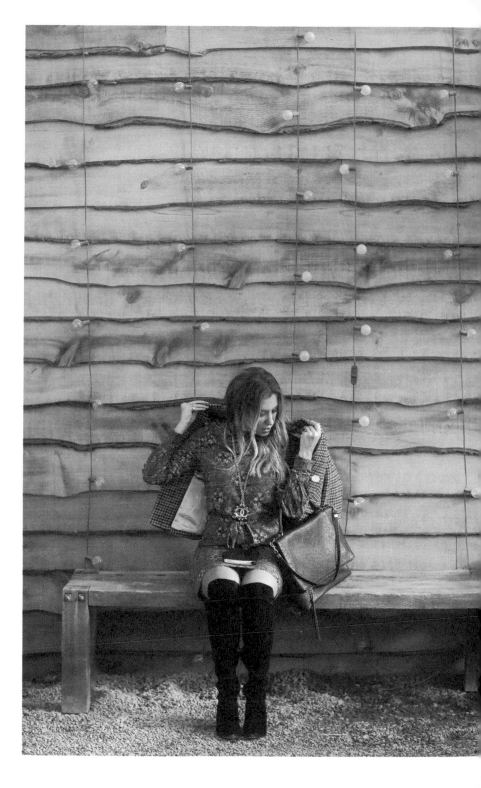

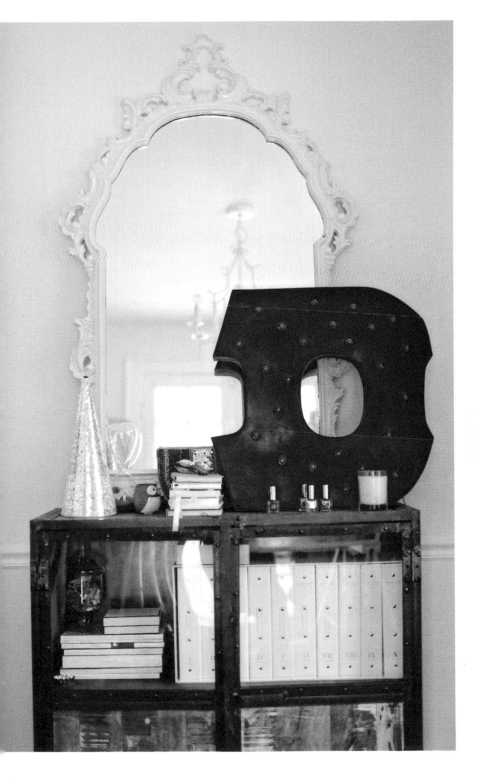

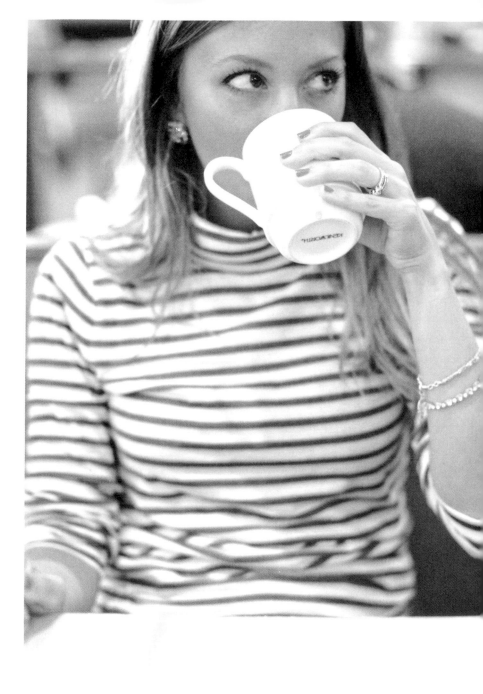

AFTERWORD

... and we meet again on the other side. Have you taken away some lessons from the book? I have. I learned that I like minimal pieces with really unique details, worn with tons of accessories. I like ladylike dresses and boho touches. I learned that I live in a fashion category of my own, and I'm proud of that.

what comes next?

You've come a long way. It's time to begin living your brand. I'd advise continuing to challenge yourself by setting new goals moving forward. Don't forget, you can always come back to this book when you are in need of some seasonal inspiration or if you want to revisit any challenges in a braver category. Only you can decide where your new look and newfound confidence can take you from here. See you at NYFW!

but Dallas, please don't go—i still have questions!

Feel free to get in touch on my social channels with any questions as you go.

dallasshaw.com
instagram.com/dallasshaw
facebook.com/DallasShaw
twitter: @dallasshaw
pinterest.com/dallasshaw

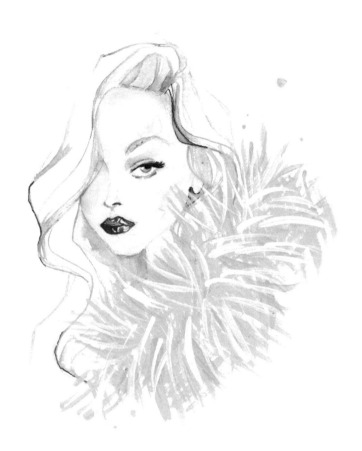

ACKNOWLEDGMENTS

{STREET CREDS}

Thanks to you for reading along. Thank you to Cara Bedick, my first editor, who helped bring the book's early vision into being, and Cassie Jones, for enthusiastically seeing it through to publication. To my agent, Caryn Karmatz Ruby, for believing in this book years before it came to be. To Kylie, the art log wizard. To my patient husband, Harold, for his logic, and to my amazing family and friends, for helping me along with this exciting process and creative endeavor.

{CREDITS}

Photos by Alison Conklin
Styling by Beka Rendell
Florals: Sullivan Owen
Summer hair: Sarah Potempa
Special Locations: Terrain,
Valley Forge Flowers

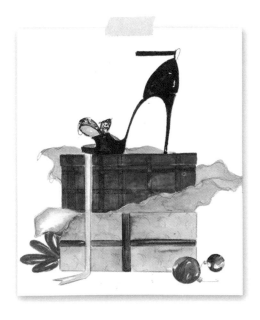

shop on, friends

3 Potato 4
AERIN
AHAlife
Angela Roi
Anthropologie Home
Antik Batik
Arielle Gordon
Arik Kastan
Australia Luxe
Banana Republic
bareMinerals
BaubleBar
Beachwaver
Bellocq Tea Atelier
BHLDN
Bibi van der Velden
Blank NYC
Brandy Pham
Brevity Jewelry
By Boe
Capezio
Christian Louboutin
Clare V.
Claudette Mar
Clé de Peau Beauté
Clyde
Colby June
COMMUNION by Joy
Crane & Canopy
Cuyana

Daniel
  Wellington
Deadly
  Ponies
Deborah
  Lippmann
Deepa
  Gurnani
Diptyque
Dolce & Gabbana
Dora Lou-Etsy
Edge O Beyond
Elina Linardaki
Elisa Solomon
Eliza Gwendalyn
Elizabeth and James
Else
Erie Basin
ERLŪM Alpaca
Essie
Estée Lauder
Eugenia Kim
Everlane
Fekkai
Fig and Yarrow
Fleur du Mal
Fleur of England
For Love and Lemons
FORESTBOUND
Fortnight Lingere

Frasier Sterling
Fresh Cosmetics
Frieda Sophie
FWRD: Else Walker
Geography 541
GiantLION
Gigi NY
Gold Silver and
  Gems—Etsy
Grace Lee
Halston
Hanky Panky
Happy Plugs
Heidi Merrick
Helen Ficalora
Herbivore Botanicals
Hourglass Cosmetics
Ivy Kirzhner
J.Crew
Jane Iredale
Jaqueline Pinto
Jennie Kwon
Jennifer Dawes Design

Jennifer Tuton
Jess Feury
Jewelera—Etsy
Journelle
JustFab
Kahina Giving Beauty
Kalmanovich
Karen Karch
Karolina Bik Jewellery
Katherine Kane
Kathryn Elyse Jewelry
Katie Carder Fine
  Jewelry (Moira Katie
  Lime)
Katie Waltman
Kenneth Cole
Kerastase
Ki-ele
KiKi Damaris
Komono
Kypris
L'Agent
La Perla
Lancôme
Laneige
Lascvicious
Le Labo
Leif Shop
Lily B and Co.
Linge Ballet
LUCA Jewelry—Etsy
Lucia Stofej Shop—Etsy
Lulu Frost
Lulus
Lumily
Mackage
Madewell
Magna Luxie
Mai Couture
Manor-Simply Smashing
  Home Decor

Marc Fisher
Marc Jacobs Beauty
Maybelline
Melissa Flagg
Michael Stars
Michele Watches
Mimi Holliday
Minnetonka
Miss Mandalay
Miu Miu
Moda Operandi
Moorea Seal
Morning Lavender
Muthology
Mullein and Sparrow
NARS
Nena and Co.
No. 2
Onata—Etsy
Otte NY
Paloma El Paso
PAUL & JOE
Pérola NYC
Perpetual Shade
Peruvian Connection
Plum Pretty Sugar
Poppin.
Prism Souls
Rab Labs
Rebecca Minkoff
Reformation
Rene Caovilla
Renee Lewis
RevitaLash
River Island
Royal Scout & Co.
Saks Fifth Avenue
Samantha Wills
Sei Swim
Seychelles Footwear
Shoe Dazzle

Shop-Skirt
Slip-Pure Silk Pillowcase
Smith & Cult
Soludos
Sorel
St. Roche
Stila
Sugar
Sunday Riley
Target
Tata Harper
Ted Baker
The Diamond Foundry
The Dreslyn
The Laundress
The Littles
The Object Enthusiast
The RealReal
TheMadRabbitShoppe—
  Etsy
Tieks
Timex
Tocca
Unearthen
Van Heesh Design
Vince Camuto
VINCE.
Volition
Waltzing Matilda
Wanderlust + Co.
WANT Les Essentiels
Warby Parker
Wild Habit
Wildfox
Work Horse Jewelry
Yosi Samra
Young NG
Zady
Zara
Zoë Chicco

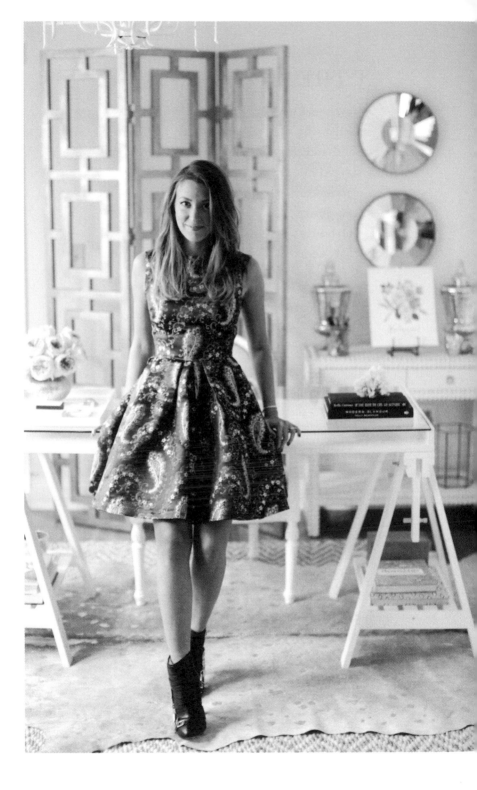

ABOUT THE AUTHOR

It was only a few short years ago that Dallas Shaw was an aspiring Disney artist who took a sharp turn on her career path, driving full speed and straight ahead toward fashion-industry royalty. She started her own business online, and now she is the most demanded fashion illustrator in the industry, acting as artist, project designer, and style ambassador to the most powerful fashion houses.

Her client list seems almost unreal. She's taken on work for Chanel, Oscar de la Renta, Ralph Lauren, Kate Spade, Dolce & Gabbana, *Harper's Bazaar*, Donna Karan, Target, Frederick Fekkai, Essie, Victoria's Secret, Nordstrom, Neutrogena, Marc Jacobs beauty, Mercedes-Benz Fashion Week, Century 21, Calypso St. Barth, Lulu Frost, Anthropologie, Free People, Ted Baker, Maybelline, Express, Coach, Joie, and more.

She's THE girl designers, beauty brands, and even travel companies call, and call back, to lend drawings and style expertise at the beginning of every important product launch. You could call her the Olivia Pope of the fashion industry. Every company knows her, every brand wants her.

She is an artist, a brand ambassador, a creative director, a boss, a TV personality, and an inspiration. In addition to her day job(s), her personal style is watched closely by 300,000 faithful fashion followers who check her social websites daily for as much art, fashion, beauty, and travel content as they can get their eyes on. In her spare time, she's pinning and tweeting all of the whimsy. She shares every moodboard, color palette, and million-dollar project online (along with the occasional joke). Followers consider Shaw their insider's secret, following her every move from the tip of her pencil to the bottoms of her Louboutins. (Yes, he's also one of her clients.)

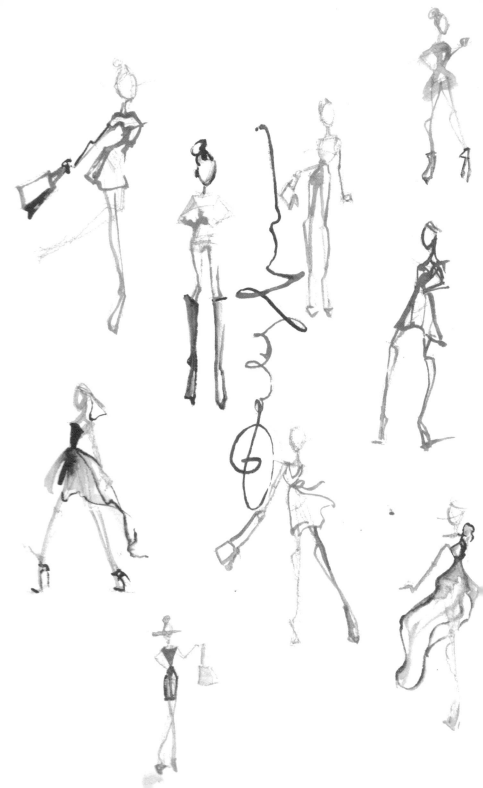